Management through the Woods and over the Rivers

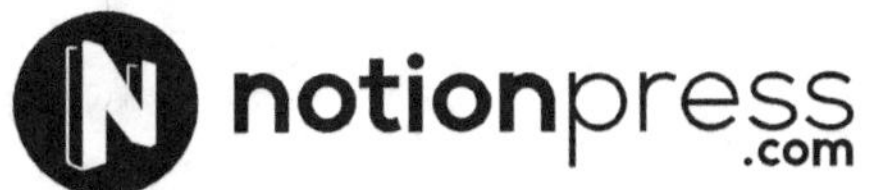

Management through the Woods and over the Rivers

Outdoor Based Experiential Training

Dr Ranjan Garge

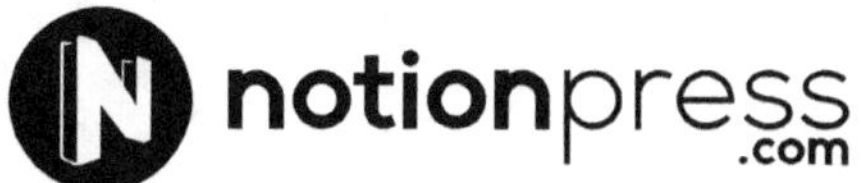

Notion Press

Old No. 38, New No. 6

McNichols Road, Chetpet

Chennai - 600 031

First Published by Notion Press 2016

Copyright © Dr Ranjan Garge 2016

All Rights Reserved.

ISBN 978-93-5206-818-0

Table of Contents

Author's note

I was introduced to Himalayan adventure through my participation in 2nd National Himalayan Trekking programme organized by Youth Hostels Association of India, New Delhi in 1969. I myself got deeply involved in Mountain adventure since 1972. By the time I did my Basic and Advance course in Mountaineering at Manali [H P] during 1972 to 74, I decided to nurture Mountaineering as my hobby. Accordingly I went on leading the Himalayan Peak Climbing expeditions, building an organization known as "Mountain Lovers association," organizing Basic and Advance Rock climbing courses in the Reserve forests in Maharashtra, and many High altitude trekking programmes in Himalaya. Being associated with education as a teacher and then the head of the educational institution as a Principal, I trained thousands of students from Dr Babasaheb Ambedkar Marathwada University, Aurangabad, Maharashtra, in Rock climbing. In 1978 I joined Youth Hostels association of India, Aurangabad chapter. Col. P N Modak, warden of the Youth Hostel was my source of inspiration. Mountain Adventure activity started spreading widely, and Youth Hostel became an approved center for Rock climbing and Mountaineering training. We started growing as a core group of Mountaineers. Side by side Industrial area around Aurangabad was also growing. In due course of time three industrial estates were established around Aurangabad with even few multinationals too.

During 90s industries in Aurangabad experienced very bad days of recession. Many industries closed down for want of modern technologies, unskilled human resource was to be replaced by skilled ones. Human resource Development in general and Soft skills in particular became a major concern for every industry. The most important change I experienced was "Focus on training and development." Old training methods were obsolete because of upcoming unpredictable industrial environment and Unforeseen situations coming in front. etc.

By the down of 21st century I had established myself as a social trainer in the Industrial estate around. I was very seriously thinking on training and development issue. Now it was an opportunity and challenge for me to think of some novel ways of training the human resource in the industrial sector. I remembered myself doing a small course in Switzerland at Basel in 1986 when I was there in connection with an academic conference. Conference management itself had given us an option for Outdoor training course of 4 days as a part of post conference activity. Being an adventurist, I did that course on a floating ship in the river. It was a wonderful experience that I ever had in my life. I started exploring and reviewing articles and research papers throughout the world on Outdoor Management concept from 1996 onwards. I started developing games and instruments required and launched an organization "COSMOS Outward Bound Pioneers" with my friends. We identified the natural spots to conduct the "Outdoor Based Experiential Training Courses" in the reserved forest near Aurangabad. Since then we have been conducting "Outdoor Based Experiential Training Programme "[OBET] in more than 20 industries in Maharashtra in an open environment at 'Patnadevi Reserve Forest,'" or Hiranya resort or Chaitanya resort in Maharashtra state. Participants included Managers, Supervisors, Workers, Principals, Teachers, Students and Support staff. In outdoors they faced the real adventure situations where the defined task is given to be completed within the constraints of Time, Resources and People.

Initially these programmes were not well received. The physical stretching and taking little risk like river crossing, rappelling or climbing a 12 feet wall was not appreciated though the safety was 100%. Many of them had seen the forests for the first time. The biggest challenge was how to translate the outdoors in to workplace situations. I new that the entire problem is related to an attitude. Since year 2000 we changed our strategy of conducting OBET courses. We concentrated more on **orientation before and in-depth evaluation after the training.** This strategy worked well. Ice breaking activities help us to relax them before confronting the task. By the year 2000 the industries in general and I T or Biotech companies in particular around the world changed their old ways of doing things. **Hierarchy** in companies diminished and **clustering** of the people as a team became a major concern. i.e. Face book, Apple, Microsoft, Banks etc. Handling unpredictable situations , Team work, Leadership and effective communication, judgment and future vision are the key areas for any industry to focus upon. Naturally Indian industries casted out their old skin and accepted the ultramodern patterns of the human resource. Indian industries started searching for new training options. OBET being the best option which evaluates the Leadership Quality, System Problem Solving ability, Experimentation, Learning from past experience, and Transferring knowledge. While going through series of situations, they were required to Analyze, Motivate,

Make judgment, Take decision, Communicate, Delegate, Plan, Use resources effectively, Lead a team, and Respond to change. Participants were evaluated from the supervisory reports, Interviews and Questionnaires before and after OBET. Results indicated that the quality decisions taken showed a direct influence on the group success. The challenging environment in the tasks, created a positive impact and high degree of awareness with potential for personal growth. The outcome of our OBET has proved to be a very effective catalyst for dynamic learning in Indian Industries and educational institutions to face the challenges of the 21st century.

It is all about making a difference:

If each grain of sand were to say;
One grain does not make a mountain,
There would be no land.

If each drop of water were to say;
One drop does not make an ocean,
There would be no sea.

If each note of music were to say;
Each note does not make a symphony,
There would be no melody.

If each word were to say;
One word does not make a book,
There would be no library.

If each brick were to say;
One brick does not make a wall,
There would be no house.

If each seed were to say;

One seed does not make a field,

There would be no harvest.

If each of us were to say;

One person does not make a difference,

There would never be love and peace on earth.

You and I do make a difference;

Begin today and make a difference.

Finally I would like to thank my guru Late Col. P N Modak, Dr M V Deshpande [Behavioral Science expert] for providing me with inspiration, Mr Prashant Deshpande [Chairman, Association of Indian Industries] for writing the foreword for this book. Forest officers of respective reserve forests for providing me the natural surrounding like reserve forests for outdoor activities, Mr Hareesh Jakhete and Sunit Athalye for providing the facilities on their resorts. I am thankful to Mountaineers Kishor Bhosale, Rafiq Shaikh and Archana Bhosale for their assistance in rope work. I am thankful to Parag pande, Maitreya Mudkavi, Chember of Marathwada Industries and Agriculture and their team for the ground support. My wife has been a constant source of motivation without which this book could not have been completed.

DR RANJAN GARGE

Email: ranjan.garge@gmail.com

Mobile : 9822634442

Foreword

Dr Ranjan Garge is a versatile professional in the field of Management. His book on Outdoor Management is on a unique and innovative subject like Outdoor Based Experiential Learning. Dr Garge is known to me over 20 years now as a management guru. In his young age he was a die-hard mountaineer and a very curious student. Being a Microbiologist, science was always core for him. He has worked in many faculties like Mountaineering, Management, Journalism, Environment and Social work. As a active Rotarian, a teacher, researcher and a science professional he has gained tremendous experience in building teams, organizing events and motivating people. He is a prolific writer with 15 books to his credit in the field of Science, Adventure and Management. His book on Mountaineering received the Best Literature award instituted by Government of Maharashtra in 1993.

I am very closely associated with his work in the field of Management development through Outdoor training methodology. In fact Dr Garge was introduced to me through such programme which was organized for my company for 20 people. This programme was organized in a Patnadevi reserved forest near Aurangabad. We spent 3 days at the forest with minimum facilities learning real life management principles. We all were mesmerized with the experience we gathered through various activities we did first time in our life. It included Physical, Mental and spiritual kind of exercises, games, situations and arrangements.

Dr Garge had designed and developed this programme very scientifically. Going to a forest and being there for 3 days was itself a mind-blowing experience. The activities like Treasure hunt, Night journey to unknown, Tiger jump, River crossing, fall of trust, Dragon walk etc. were vibrant and generated lot of curiosity. We basically learnt how to tackle the unforeseen situations. These activities removed our physical and mental blocks. These activities opened our mind to understand hidden potentials of all the members and later we were able to utilize those potentials in handling the real life challenges and workplace situations. The biggest learning was the realization of TEAM strength, members' inner potential and huge boost in self-confidence. This is a story 20 years ago and I still remember every aspect of this training programme. This programme no doubt has a long term impact.

I am glad that Dr Ranjan Garge, a man with first-hand experience in the field, has written this book. May be the first Indian writer to take a detailed account of Outdoor Management concept. It is a good compilation of theory and concepts supported by his own practical experience.

Prashant Deshpande
Managing Director,
Expert Global Solutions,
+91 9225246800

1. Understanding the relationships

Understanding relationships means that, things make sense to the learner in terms of his or her own current experience and thinking. We know well, from all the research into learner's own ideas, that they try to make sense of things around them long before we interfere to "teach" them.

Teaching for understanding:

In my long involvement in classroom and outdoor teaching – over 40 years I have seen how the things keep changing. Developments in other fields can influence the way we look at our own field of work. Literacy leads us to recognize three important aims of teaching: Teaching for understanding, Teaching for Motivation for learning and Teaching for how to learn and how to assess one's own learning (Wynne 2002). Understanding means that, things make sense to the learner in terms of his or her own current experience and thinking. We know well, from all the research into learner's own ideas that they try to make sense of things around them long before we interfere to "teach" them. When we intervene, we need to take the learner's own ideas as a starting point. This means encouraging them to test their own ideas and alternatives, so that they realize the value of more broadly applicable concept. This will only be effective if the learner knows how to collect and use evidence in relation to the phenomena they are studying by applying appropriate enquiry skills.

Motivation for learning:

Motivation is a complex concept and it has many shades of meaning. A learner can be motivated by interest and enjoyment in finding things out. A learner can also be motivated by fear and punishment or by a prospect of a reward. These different kinds of motivations have apro found impact on learning. If a child is motivated by interest in enjoyment then it is called **"INTRINSIC"** motivation. It means that there is a satisfaction in learning. Learner will persist with it., engage in future learning and not be satisfied until it is understood. Intrinsically motivated leads to higher levels of achievements and is described as **"DEEP"** as against **"SURFACE"** learning. Second type of motivation is called **"EXTRINSIC."** Learner here is engaged in their task mainly because of external incentives. It leads to learning that is undertaken as quickly as possible and with minimum efforts to gain the rewards., whether it is praise or passing a test. This tends to encourage shallow or surface learning. Here learners focus their attention on memorizing the facts and mastering the routine skills without understanding, and forgetting them soon after the test has been passed. The third type of motivation is **"ACHIEVEMENT MOTIVATION,"** influence those who strive hard to be top in the merit list, succeed by sheer efforts and find their rewards in comparing themselves with others.

Emphasizing learning goals:

Let us understand first why are we doing something and more likely to be motivated to do it if we know that what our goal is. So when thetrainees are embarking on a learning activity it is important for them to know what they are aiming for in terms of learning. Often they are told what they are to **do** but not what they will be **learning.** There is considerable evidence that the more trainees are involved in knowing the goals of their activities the more likely it is that their efforts and motivation are enlisted. Thus if we want them to focus on their learning it is important to communicate learning goals rather than performing goals. More over their energy is more likely to be directed towards developing enquiry skills and big ideas.

Learning how to learn and assess their own learning:

Encouraging trainees to think the way they do things and to reflect on their own thinking is introducing them to meta-cognition. When we are conscious of doing something grand reflect on its value. We are more likely to apply that kind of thinking again in a future situation where it is relevant. The involvement of trainees in assessing their own learning both requires and encourages them to reflect on learning.

* The assessment is used by trainers to adapt training.

* Trainers give feedback to trainees in terms of how to improve their work, not in terms of judgmental comments, grades or marks.

* Trainees are actively engaged in learning – meaning that they are active in developing their understanding and not passively receiving information.

* The trainees are engaged in self-assessment and in helping to decide their next steps.

* The trainer regards all the trainees as being capable of learning.

Indian schools:

It has been a matter of experience that learning in Indian atmosphere is based on **Extrinsic motivation**. There is a demand for more transparent and reliable system of examination, evaluation and reporting. Examinations primarily test the memory of learners and does not promote creativity among them. Learning in Indian atmosphere gives emphasis on predictability. Since the pattern of the question paper is fixed and unchanged, learning simply involves absorbing the past. Such system is effective in the environment that is stable and predictable. No such predictability and stability exists today. In the era of Liberalization, Privatization and Globalization, the world has become more interconnected. Available information and knowledge also is changing vary fast. In this situation learning process becomes more dynamic and complex. In fact the whole education system must become **"Learningful."** It means encouraging learner to think about the way they do things and reflecting on the sort of thinking they have been engaged in, to bring it to the front of their consciousness (Adey 1997). It has considerable value for life long learning. If the educational institutions in India have to truly excel in future, they will have to discover how to tap learners' and teachers' commitment and capacity to learn at all levels in the organization. In this study I have designed a continuous improvement programme which is aimed at achieving newer heights of effectiveness and capability of students and teachers. The central issue often lost sight of and seldom recognized is that, all the for going processes are possible where there is within the organization a commitment to learning. How can the education improve without first learning something new? Solve the problem?

Experimenting? Developing a new model? Re-engineering a learning process? All this require seeing a world in a new light and acting accordingly. In the absence of learning, individuals simply repeat old practices. In the process of education; policy makers, Directorate of education, Principal, Teachers, Students and non-teaching staff all are deeply involved. It is no longer sufficient to have one person or a small group of persons learning for the organization. Education policy must emphasize thinking, experimenting and most important is responding proactively to ever-changing environment, asking right questions, refine new ideas continually. We implemented a model of "Outdoor Based Experiential Training Programme" [OBET] to catalyze the process of learning in more than twenty companies in Maharashtra. Sample data of following five companies in Aurangabad city, Maharashtra state, India like 1. Expert Global Solutions Pvt. Ltd. 2. Man Diesel. 3. Sanjeev Auto 4. S S Controls 5. Aurangabad Electricals has been presented as a case study. **"COSMOS Outward Bound Pioneers, India"** [NGO] conducted OBET programme for these companies in an open environment like Reserve Forest, or resorts at various places in Maharashtra.

2. Experiential training works magic!

How do abseiling, mountain climbing, Jungle trekking, river crossing improve management skills? When confronted with OMD, skeptics can leave the accusation that the tasks required of the participants are much irrelevant than the tasks they would be faced with at a work based course. However as training concentrates on team building, Outdoor management Development plays an increasing role.

The last 40 years has seen a rapid evolution of Outdoor Management Development [OMD] as a valid and successful means of training managers, teams and leaders. This originates from the willingness by an increasing number of companies to recognize the need of personal development among their employees. It is allied to the growing perception that managers need not only learn professional and technical skills but also leadership skills. i.e. the skills to delegate, to build teams, to motivate and so on.

Initially the OMD was acknowledged as a powerful means of developing leaders, but the courses were not tailored. There was very little preparation done before hand between the buyer and the provider and there was almost no follow-up afterwards at the workplace. The courses might work or may not. The means of integrating the courses with the workplace to make sure that the lessons learned stayed learned was not there. Nowadays however, the buyers of

OMD courses often want those courses to play an important part in long lasting change.

Therefore the courses increasingly have a longer preparation time, the results are measured and the courses are followed up at the workplaces. The provider of OMD now deals in providing packages which are purposely designed to meet specific client objective.

How OMD works?

It is widely accepted that one of the most effective and powerful methods of learning is by experience. This is often difficult to supply in indoor work based training where trial and error is difficult to encourage and any experience to be gained comes from fairly obvious imitations of work-based situations.

OMD is a method of training which uses the outdoors as a context for providing real experiences., the benefits of which can then be translated back in to the workplace through frequent and detailed analytical review.

The procedure followed is as follows.

Do ---------------→ Review ------------→ Apply ------------→ Do

The difference between the OMD and work based methods of training is sharply evident. There are obvious advantages to be gained from each and for this reason OMD providers insist that their training should be seen in the context of the whole training programme for a particular company. I personally feel that The advantages of OMD are that, however relevant a work based course may seem, training in the outdoor, away from the pressures and inhibitions of work, using new, strange and real situations which demand real and original solutions can be a far more powerful experience and one which will make a much greater impact on that person, therefore causing a real and long lasting retention.

The outdoors are used because

- The task and the problems are real. The quality of decisions taken will have a clear and direct influence on the group's success.
- The new environment creates a receptiveness towards learning.
- There is a great deal of scope for working in group and need to co-operate with others to be successful.
- A challenging environment creates a positive impact and a high degree of awareness with tremendous potential for personal growth.

Companies use OMD in four main areas

- Leadership development.
- Team building 1. Rebuilding existing teams 2. Building new teams 3. Teaching team skills.
- Supporting organization development schemes. With the increase in the implementation of Total Quality Management programme the changes in management and team structure can be clearly illustrated to the workforce through OMD.
- Cross-cultural training. This frequently takes place between two companies merging or between the branches of the same company in different countries or areas.

Preparation:

As can be seen from the range of aims, the objectives of the company who send their delegates on OMD courses need to be specific and focused. The majority of tailored courses are designed after careful consultation between the provider and the buyer. Often this consultation and course preparation can last between six to nine months and can involve pre course analysis of the participants by the provider.

This detailed attitude to the preparation of courses is important because, to be successful, the courses must reflect the company culture, meet the specific corporate objectives and address the personal development of the individual delegate.

Thus with the growing sophistication of the field, the buyer of the OMD course must have clear, specific objectives and must understand where the OMD course will fit in to his company's training programme. Examples of the kind of objectives set for a course could read as follows. "Through practical experience of real situations the course should increase the ability and knowledge of the participants in the following areas: Team work, Team leadership, Styles of Management, Individual self-development and giving and receiving the feedback."

As the preparation before courses become increasingly developed, the follow-up afterwards is also increasing in importance. This usually takes the form of individual action plans, prepared by the trainers and the individual participants.

Tailored vs open courses:

OMD providers generally offer a variety of tailor-made and open courses. Each has its advantages. The open courses mean that a small number of staff can get the benefit of OMD relatively cheaply, there is healthy mixture of organizations, job levels,and personalities. It also means there is greater confidentiality for the participants. However open courses also mean that there can be no team building on permanent basis; the participants only learn about his/herself and receives no input or support from other members of their organization. Also open courses are not specifically designed for that particular individual and do not take in to account the characteristics of that person's company and therefore cannot be so relevant or effective as tailored courses.

Those companies which choose tailored courses are usually looking for long lasting change across the whole organization and as such their courses are designed to respond to real and clearly established needs and to be suitable for each of the participants chosen to attend the course.

Content of courses:

Courses can last for weekends or for a week. At impact the average size of the course is 20 and this group will then have two trainers and four backup staff working with them. Courses can be made up of whole department or a cross company vertical slice which covers all departments and all levels.

The courses will vary but the general format will consist of practical exercises, whether indoors or outdoors, followed by the sessions of review and feedback. Where the trainers and participants will draw the comparisons between the processes used in the exercises and the same processes used in very different circumstances in the workplace. In most cases task increase in complexity as the course progresses but providers usually spend approximately the last quarter of each course on review.

Most courses are progressive so that the participants can learn from mistakes. Physical aspects can also be varied as can the amount of use which is made of the outdoors. It is really up to the buyer to have the course constructed to meet their needs and suit their delegates.

Real situations:

As we saw earlier one of the main advantages of OMD is that the participants face real situations which require the group to act as a team and the leader for a particular task to use a whole range of management skills to get the task done. Thus at some stage of the course the participants are required to: Analyze and carefully examine the information, Convince, Research, Motivate/encourage and support, consult, Make judgments, Take decisions, Communicate, Plan, Monitor, Budget, Control/expedite, Report, Use resources effectively, Lead a team, and Respond to change.

Skepticism:

When confronted with OMD, skeptics can leave the accusation that the tasks required of the participants are much irrelevant than the tasks they would be faced with at a work based course. For instance they could question the relevance of delegates having to "buy" suitable equipment, collect various items from the widespread area, abseil down the cliff, build a raft. Although such a programme is a game, when the team is standing at the top of the cliff the situation is very real and at that moment the individuals concerned do need leadership. They do have to act as a team and the leader has to make real decisions. Communicate them well, delegate to his team and motivate them to carry out the task successfully.

Experiences such as this are made more valuable by the review sessions immediately afterwards where the trainers can comment on the performance of the individuals and the group and lead them in to realizing that the processes they used during the exercise were in fact the same processes as used by managers, teams and individuals at their workplace. This fact should not be lost on the participants themselves who will develop in self-awareness throughout the course owing to the nature of the challenges they will face and the feedback they will be given.

Wide range of opportunities:

Training outdoors open up a new range of opportunities. OMD strips away details of work-based knowledge leaving the delegates and trainers free to focus on good leadership, management and team skills. Because of the nature of the tasks, OMD ensures that all delegates have to actively participate.

With high professional operations all the activities have been thought through with the client to ensure that the team, leadership and the management processes used in each task are relevant and easily transferred back to workplace.

Indications show that financial sector organizations are making more and more use of OMD, to satisfy their need to train teams and leaders. Those organizations which are implementing Total Quality Management programmes have found OMD particularly useful as an established long term element in their training and development schemes.

3. Pedagogy: Do – Review – Apply – Do

Outdoor training is not about outdoor pursuits. It is a means by which the challenge, the novelty and physical reality of the environment and the skills needed to deal with it are harnessed to help managers develop other skills directly relevant to their jobs. Individuals may indeed enjoy the satisfaction that comes from doing things that they have never experienced before. Management development is not a training course or set of development exercises. It is part and parcel of enabling people to identify the work that has to be done and helping them to evolve a process of working together to achieve that work given the differences that will exist between them.

I am not going on an assault course!

I had enough of that sort of thing in the army!

Oh yes! I know, I did an outward Bound course when I was eighteen...

Sure! We send our managers...

Comments like this illustrate the problems that management development and training approaches which use the outdoors have to overcome if they are to be understood and properly used. Because the physical aspect of this type of training is exiting, the underlying issues for trainers – what it can and cannot do, the questions that need to be considered if it is to be used effectively – have received less serious attention leading to a risk that a variety of current activities and their potential for developing managers is obscured behind vivid publicity. Pictures of men and women climbing a cliff faces, trekking across the mountain convey the image. But they do less than justice to the serious intent that can underlay the activities.

Of course, some conventional approaches can be effective; for example, where a particular subject has to be learnt that directly relates to the manager's job, such as financial or planning technique. However, classroom approaches to the demands of the broader management role do seem inadequate when dealing with issues related to the manager's actual behavior.

Managers can easily rationalize a lake of success as a "fault in the rules" or claim that, "I would act differently in a real situation." In so doing they can avoid facing up to their own performance – failing to convince their colleagues of the wisdom of their proposals or failing to act decisively when faced with a number of options.

Our own work over the past 20 years in the use of the outdoor environment for management development is largely based on these ideas. While the approach adopted with different companies is varied. The essence is that managers have to **act** in a real situation which can then be **reviewed** to help them **learn** about and modify their behavior.

Managers apply their skills to a range of tasks which are quite different to those they face at work, but which are challenging and real. The results of their action are immediately apparent, providing clear evidence of their performance and a basis for feedback, questioning and experiment. Although the outdoor tasks are not **normal** they are inescapably **real.** Managing an outdoor situation is like managing life. It is full of unpredictable events and people. Result has to be achieved with only limited resources and time available.

In this situation any decision to act outside an agreed overall plan results in a group being in the wrong place at the wrong time- a clear lesson on the consequences of committing resources without adequate communication.

A failure to communicate clearly within a group will reveal itself quickly and as different understanding of a method of tackling a task show themselves in confusions, diversions and frustrations.

Because the tasks are physically real, and stretch a group in terms of time and space, all participants need to contribute and there are less chances of an individual participant avoiding issues as he might in the classroom situation, by staying in the background or by role playing. In short space of time many critical incidents occur, continuously confronting the manager with the result of his performance, and in total providing an intense, clear and potent means of learning.

OMD Programmes are vivid and engaging and everyone is fully involved, *but not necessarily all doing the same things* and it inculcates a pattern of involuntary learning that means people can't help but get involved and learn and take away useful lessons and insights. At the simplest level, outdoor training is fun and a great way to get to know & understand people better. For new teams and newly appointed managers there are many lessons that can be learned quickly. At best a good programme can really accelerate the learning process considerably and speed up the development of a wide range of management and team working process skills.

Hiranya Resort, which is situated at the foot hills of Daulatabad fort near Aurangabad, Maharashtrais or other training ground like reserve forests, where we have the means through various activities to heighten people's emotional states through exciting and challenging activities. Other means might involve a time limit or multiple tasking. This can make a leader's job much harder during an exercise. And of course doing a task underground or on water or on the edge of a cliff may also heighten the pulse rate. In our experience people revertwhen under mild stress, and this is a useful phenomenon which can be used in a good humored way to help discuss and reflect on leadership styles, decision-making processes, efficientteam working methods, communications, delegation, etc.

At a higher level, outdoor based training may be able to afford delegates to give insights and changes in attitudes and behavior patterns that may not be so easily or safely inculcated or fed back to people so effectively in their normal work environment. I frequently point out to clients that we are not "experts" in outdoor training, but we do have many years of experience of providing clients with appropriate ***"open forums"*** for colleagues in real teams to exchange of ideas, beliefs, values, and to heighten sensitivity of other people's problems, etc. Being in a strange new environment often helps strip away rank, clannish feelings, assumptions and prejudices, and can generate a real feeling of fellowship with a sense of openness, care and a willingness to help each other that is hard to describe in words to one who hasn't experienced the feeling. Residential programme also helps clients get away from the ringing telephones and "chill-out" away from other distractions.

A change can be as good as a rest and this is particularly valuable for cross-functional team development when lots of little teams need to start working as a more cohesive to enable cultural change, continuous improvement, implementation of Kaizen philosophy and so on. I wonder how many firms are out there where their senior managers keep saying they'd like to see their teams working more closely together?

OMD is activity based:

1. One activity is more worthwhile than another if it **permits** delegates to make **informed choices** in carrying out the activity and the opportunity to **reflect on the consequences** of their choices.

2. One activity is more worthwhile than another if it assigns learners **active roles** in the learning situation rather than passive ones.

3. One activity is more worthwhile than another if it asks learner to engage in **inquiry of ideas**, applications of intellectual processes or current problems either personal, social or work-related.

4. One activity is more worthwhile than another if it involves students with **real** objects, materials, data or artifacts.

5. One activity is more worth while than another if the completion of a task can be accomplished successfully by learners of different fitness at several **different levels of ability**, if necessary with some inputs from Directing Staff.

6. One activity is more worthwhile than another if it challenges learners to examine **in a new setting** an

idea, an application of an intellectual process, or a current **problem** which has not been previously studied.

7. One activity is more worthwhile than another if it requires students to examine topics or issues that citizens in our society do not normally examine – and that are typically ignored by the major communications media in our nation.

8. One activity is more worthwhile than another if it involves learners and tutors in "risk taking" – not a risk of life and limb – but a **risk of success or failure**.

9. One activity is more worthwhile than another if it requires students to **rewrite**, **rehearse** and **polish** their initial efforts.

10. One activity is more worthwhile than another if it involves learners in the application and mastery of **meaningful rules** and standards or disciplines.

11. One activity is more worthwhile than another if it gives students the chance to **share in the planning, the carrying out of a plan**, or the results of an interesting and engaging **activity** with others.

12. One activity is more worthwhile than another if it **is relevant to the expressed training needs, interests** and purposes of the learners.

13. An activity which inculcates the desired outputs and effects enjoyably in a **shorter time** than others activities which probably is going to be more useful to the delegates than activities which take up lots of time.

14. Activities packed into programmes which are too short a duration (say at the client's request) may

be far less effective in providing useful forums for open discussion than activities within more realistic programmes of a slightly longer duration.

Spectrum of activities:

It appears to us that there is a spectrum of activities using the outdoor environment, all of which may be appropriate for particular needs. At one end of the spectrum is the event which offers a strong physical bias, a high element of individual development of outdoor pursuit's skills and little direct relevance to organizational/management development needs. However it may offer the individual an opportunity for self-discovery and a chance to develop a higher level of awareness of his impact on others outside the normal working situation. Moving across the spectrum there are events which utilize a certain level of outdoor skills, applied to the completion of the group tasks, giving opportunities to explore managerial skills of leadership and communication. Towards the other end of the spectrum one can also find organizations running events which do not demand specific outdoor skills but which do demand that participants accomplish real tasks in real environment, perhaps using their past experience to construct a bridge or to negotiate an obstacle. Such an event is a more vivid version perhaps of the classroom situation where constructional games involving planning and action are well established in the management skills and communication area.

Our outdoors have involved us in observing or using activities at various points on this spectrum. We have particularly sought to explore and add to the element of "Managing uncertainties" in our own events of managers. to go beyond the defined tasks that develops skills appropriate to the leadership of a group with a clear problem to salve. We have sought to create tasks that demand first a clarification of objectives and of alternative solutions, then appropriately co-ordinate activity.

Given such a varied range of activities it is clear that the trainer suggesting or arranging an outdoor event needs to consider carefully

- The objectives of the activity for a group or individual involved.

- Suitability of the particular methods adopted by the organization offering the activity or with whom he intends to work.

The pattern of event:

We found that there are two strands to consider in planning the event.

- **The intellectual and emotional strand**, concerned with developing participant's awareness or managerial/organizational issues and their own skills and behavior.

- **The physical strand**, concerned with developing the raw material of experience on which the participants can reflect and on which the tutors can base their own contributions.

Since we have approached the use of the outdoors as management Development specialists and not as outdoors pursuits specialists we have found that the first stand must be the primary concern. Physical activities can then be related to it, which in our opinion is secondary.

In order to develop the intellectual strand we have found it helpful to recognize that managers have to cope with working situations which can be classified according to the degree of familiarity of the problem and its method of solution.

Problem solving

In Box 1 are the simple problems – the problem itself is clear. The way of dealing with it is known. The experienced manager deals with such a problem almost automatically, given that he has been taught the correct problem solving technique. In Box 2 the problem itself is still clear, but the method of solution is unfamiliar and demands thought and perhaps a measure of creativity on the part of those seeking to solve the problem. In Box 3 and 4 the problem itself becomes less clear. There are alternative ways of defining the problem. Perhaps as the situation moves from Box 1 to Box 4 the manager is faced with increasing demands of insight, creativity and skills in dealing with other people and so on. For more junior and middle managers the major part of their organizational life may have been concerned with dealing with Box 1 and Box 2 problems. As they move to higher levels of the organization the situation they face are not dealt with on the straight forward application of techniques in accordance with established practice. They have to cope with ambiguity and uncertainty and with conflicting views on the definition of the problem and on ways of tackling it.

One of the major management development problems to be faced is thus the need to convert the manager from a problem solver to an opportunity seeker, taking a broad view of alternative courses of action open to him and accepting that new situations create unfamiliar demands and that he has to work through complex processes to identify and implement an effective response, recognizing that there may be no one right solution.

Using this framework the pattern of an event can be developed, task being made progressively more complex and demanding. Early in the event relatively simple tasks with clear results can be used... Such task might involve the crossing of a designated obstacle using an assortment of planks, drums and ropes without any one touching the ground with in the time constraint. Such exercise can be useful in developing the participants skills of communication and in beginning to explore group issues related to trust and conflict.

As the event progresses more complex tasks with more open objectives and more varied constraints can be introduced to reflect the movement from Box 1 to Box 4. We have found that a deliberate qualitative design shift is needed. It is not enough to simply expand the task – to make it bigger by adding a lot of Box 1 problems together in the sequence, which may do no more than provide more individuals with opportunities to take leadership role or practice particular communication skills.

Thus our events have evolved to include final exercises that have deliberately contained choices of objectives.

* Do we concentrate on finding this objective?
* Or on finding a person who put it in place?
* Or on mapping the total situation and trying to do both?
* How can we deploy our resources given that we appear to have several courses of action to pursue simultaneously?

These are the sorts of questions that a group has to face as it confronts the later stages of an event and the Box 4 problems. Obviously, the intellectual strand of an event has to concern itself with more than the categorization of the tasks to be undertaken. From the designers point of view it provides a way of building up the pattern of tasks and is one useful framework for reviewing those tasks as the event progresses. For the participants the major component of the intellectual strand is their own experience of the tasks and the lesson derived from review of that experience.

Thus there is a need for a framework against which the participants can review their performance. We have found that the best approach here is to use the managers' own prior knowledge and experience. Thus at start of the event ask them to state their own "principles of management." Most will produce the conventional list – e.g. Define the problem, plan, delegate, co-ordinate, communicate, monitor etc.

As the event progresses this list is used as a review framework, building up to embrace far more than the original in two respects.

Firstly it quickly becomes evident that the theory that the list represents frequently does not accord with actual behavior when faced with the task., and a new list emerge that is more specific in relation to what the manager actual has to do to cope adequately with the situation.

Secondly, the skills area comes to the force, reflecting the difference between knowing about principles of management and actual possessing the skills needed to implement those principles in a face to face situation.

Experiential cycle:

The event thus follows an experiential cycle, each task experience being reviewed to produce new insights in to effective managerial behavior. As the event progresses tutors may introduce other relevant frameworks to help the group to clarify what it has learnt. Such inputs may embrace concepts of team development, connected issues of inter-personal relationships, individual/organizational balances, process/task balances and so on. There does not seem to have any definite order for such inputs, it is a matter of judgment as the event progresses and the need of the group and the individuals become clear.

Some issues for using the outdoors:

Our experience suggests that there are four key areas to consider when using the outdoor approach.

1. Briefing and pre-event activity
2. Event design
3. Tutorial resources
4. Follow up activity.

Briefing and pre-event activity is the biggest determinant of eventual effectiveness. It is particularly important because of the misunderstanding and false impression that both the participants and their organization may have about this form of activity. Accordingly we recommend discussion of individual learning aims and comprehensive briefing before the event. – not only on the level of learning objectives but also personal level – to reassure participants about physical fitness, clothing, equipment's, insurance etc. Accommodation can be worry, particularly for sr. Managers. and Government officers. So the aim is participants should arrive at the event with a clear idea of the particular areas they would like to develop. E.g. Strategic planning skills, capacity to co-ordinate groups, to tackle unforeseen situations. They should also have a reasonable idea of what to expect, and be reassured that the event will not present impossible physical challenges or compulsory risk taking. They should be adequately briefed about the clothing and accommodation.

Design of event presents several issues for the trainer. We have found that flexibility is vital if people of different ages, aptitudes and skills are to be allowed full opportunities to be involved and to contribute and practice the skills most relevant to each individual. So we have tried to ensure that the event does not impose set demands on the participants by requiring that a certain number of people be trained to a given level of competence in a particular skill and then presenting a clearly defined task demanding that those specific skills be utilized.

We have found great value in allowing all participants to acquire some new skills relevant to the outdoor tasks.

When the group has identified the roles to be performed and allocated them to members. Some may then undertake predominantly physical role, others may be processing data, others planning and co-coordinating the overall effort of the group. All members of a group should have an opportunity to acquire and thus to use, novel outdoor skills such as basic navigation or rope work. It is up to the individual and the group to utilize total resources most effectively. To us this seems to maximize the opportunities for valuable learning in the area of decision making, role allocation and resource utilization.

Flexibility applies to other aspects of the design:

Timings: Given the varying needs of different groups and individual, the sequence of exercises and inputs seems highly time flexible.

Physical pitch: Readiness to vary the level of demands to match the capacity of individuals and groups seems most important.

Leadership and competition: In none of the events we actually appoint a leader – although we have been involved in events where the skills of leading a group have been a focus of attention. Our experience suggests that to allocate the role of leader to one member of a group can run counter to the dynamics of the group, whether the group consists of colleagues from one organization or comparative strangers. The functions of leadership and the relative issues of the leader's skills and how the group reacts are for us integral with other aspects of the event. We have found this approach relevant to most managers working in complex organizations where leadership is often distributed and transient. Deliberately creating competition between teams does not seem to us to be helpful in itself as a design feature. We have found that dividing participants in to sub groups, especially for the earlier part of the event, can help learning, by allowing for close exploration of individual needs and work on basic skills. As more complex exercises are undertaken, the inter-action and co-operation of such "teams" can also be valuable for development of strategic co-ordination and communication skills.

However to set up deliberate competition throughout an event seems to us likely to create the risk that winning team will see their success as evidence of satisfactory performance than possibly the result of facing incompetent opposition! We have found that objectives set in relation to the team's own standards or targets set by the tutors are more helpful than beating the competing teams when seeking to achieve development based on review of performance during a task.

The third key area is the role and competence of the **Tutorial team**. The tutors have to be able to combine to achieve the right balance between the intellectual and the physical. It is important to draw out the industrial, organizational and personal relevance of the experience and this requires both process skills and ability to provide relevant inputs. The more one is seeking to use the outdoors as a means rather than an end, the more important this tutor role becomes. Without industrial experience and relevance, these events are simply hiding behind the mountains.

Instructors have to balance challenge and risk with safety and awareness of the stress that the novelty of the outdoors can produce. To be effective they also have to stand back and allow the participants to generate ideas, solve problems and apply their skills... We also have found that technically simple problems can be very effective and that technical complexity – more outdoor equipment and more specialized skills and roles – does not necessarily help learning.

Lastly we see **Follow up** as a critical issue. All training events involve this, but in case of outdoor events we feel there are particular dangers. In a way these are mirror images of those we seek to guard against by proper briefing.

There is a danger that on return to the organization the participant will encounter a lake of understanding from bass and colleagues that is heightened by their misconceptions about this form of activity, and that accordingly the participants experience and learning is not reinforced. This is one reason why we feel that a team oriented approach or an event involving participants from the same parent organization, offers the best chance of effective follow up.

4. Learning to learn by doing

In my own Forty years of experience in using the outdoors with managers, I have found the review of the processes involved in physical activities to be a constituent element of outdoor development. Without it, the learning is haphazard; the benefits are left to chance. I use adventures purely as an educational vehicle....Dr Ranjan Garge.

...What is outdoor development and how does it fit into traditional management development? Outdoor development may be very adventurous to the participants who stretch themselves in the challenging activities, yet it is not adventure in the usual meaning of the word.

"To me adventure involves a journey, or a sustained Endeavour, in which there are the elements of risk and of the unknown which have to be overcome by the physical skills of the individual." Wrote mountaineer **Chris Bonington.** "Furthermore an adventure is something that an individual chooses to do and where the risk involved is self-imposed and threatens no one but himself." **Colin J. Mortlock** defines adventure education as that which uses as a medium those outdoor pursuits which are potentially dangerous. It involves the presentation of a meaningful challenge to people within a framework of safety, in order to give them a deep personal and social awareness. The emphasis in such an approach is on the individual and the focus is on the physical task rather than on a management development, organization need, or on the process people go through in outdoor development actives.

The adventure, **John Ridgway**, who rowed across the Atlantic with Chay Blyth in 1966, has conducted adventure courses for managers. When asked by one of his clients, IBM, to incorporate debriefings and discussions, about processes that accompanied thephysical tasks, he simply declined to do them or to allow IBM trainers to carry them out feedback and analysis during the course itself. Review of the adventure activities is down to the individuals in their own time after the outdoor programmers.

In my own forty years of experience in using the outdoors with managers, I have found the review of the processes involved in physical activities to be a constituent element of outdoor development. Without it, the learning is haphazard; the benefits are leftto chance. My own use of adventures is purely as an educational vehicle, as part of anintegrated programme of activities which present frequent opportunities for reflection on experiences and situations occurring within the course, in an effort to realize specific objectives in relation to the individual's personal development and the work situation.

"The Leadership Trust" over its nine-year history has put greater emphasis on course review and process analysis of its physical activities, cutting back on these activities to provide more rooms for real learning. The Leadership Trust, for example, no longer runs all-nights exercises because these left the men too tired to concentrate on the learning.

Without built–in debriefings to get at the transferable learning and valuable lessons inherent in physical tasks in the outdoors, a programme could become a purely personal adventure.

Expedition to Kilimanjaro!

The dangerous sports club begun at oxford in the late 1970s, for example had personal impact and value akin to outdoor development programmers for some of its participants. Simon, one of the club's members, described an expedition the club made in 1979 to hang-glide from the 19,340 feet high summit of Kilimanjaro. At the end of his report, he observed that had the event been an outdoor development programme for managers.

1. A firm's money, not his own, would have been at risk;

2. The activity would have been better scheduled and more tightly organized with a permit to use the mountain obtained beforehand and

3. The group would have been accompanied by experts in mountaineering and hang – gliding.

The young manager's observation about the risk being diminished by outdoor development is quite correct; however, his supposition that this would have devalued the experience is open to question. On the contrary, a systematic outdoor development may well have made the Kilimanjaro expedition the learning experience of a lifetime.

The essential difference between adventure and out-door development, then, is that in adventure the activity is primary and any learning that results is by product whereas, in outdoor development, the physical event is subordinate to the primary activity, which is the learning about leadership, team building communications, one self, others, stress management, decision making etc.

In the outdoor development programmes the essential characteristics of outdoor development are the use of outdoors, incorporation of process reviews and application of experiential learning methods.

Management development for "real"

'Management development for real' is.

1. To provide knowledge of theory, best practice technologies and techniques.

2. To foster appropriate positive attitudes; and

3. To develop practical specific skills.

The traditional way of imparting knowledge through lectures, readings, assignments, discussions, tests, etc. Are well tried in schooling and form a normal part of management education. Case studies add a new dimension for knowledge transmission. But attitudinal change is often needed if a manager is to act in harmony with the knowledge of management science. A set of attitude is required for managers which includes self-confidence, trust in colleagues, a participative exercise of authority, a readiness to act, a willingness to lead and inspire team work the capability to change, the eagerness to take responsibility and the ability to delegate. These types of attitudes are shaped by positive and powerful emotional experiences which are fostered by interpersonal activities.

Experiential learning, then, becomes a vital component of effective management development. It is a process 'which begins with the experience, followed by reflection, discussions, analysis and evaluation of the experience. The assumption is that we seldom learn from experience unless we assess the experience, assigning our own meaning in terms of our own goals, aims, ambitions and expectations'.

It is precisely such an experiential learning model that is used in outdoor development. The circular learning pattern developed by **Kolb** and shown in **Figure 1** is appropriate as model for learning in outdoor development.

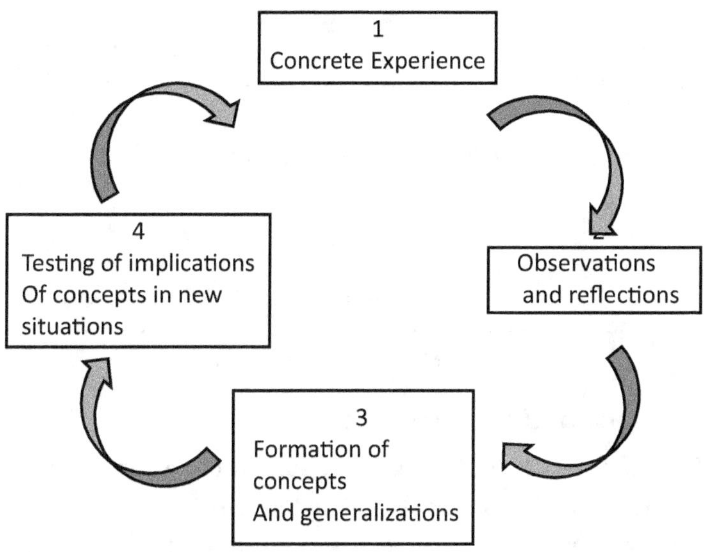

Figure 1 : Circular Learning Pattern

Further linking into how outdoor Development fits into a managerial skills framework can be gathered from **Waters'** analysis of Marginal skill Development as shown in **Figure 2**. Outdoor development would fit into the classification he labels **insight skills** which include working in groups, dealing with ambiguity and change, building trust and negotiating. **Context skill** include goal setting, work planning, designing controls, building commitment. **Wisdom** embraces: charisma, entrepreneurship, strategy formulation, Finally, **Practical skill** include performance appraising, report writing, active listening.

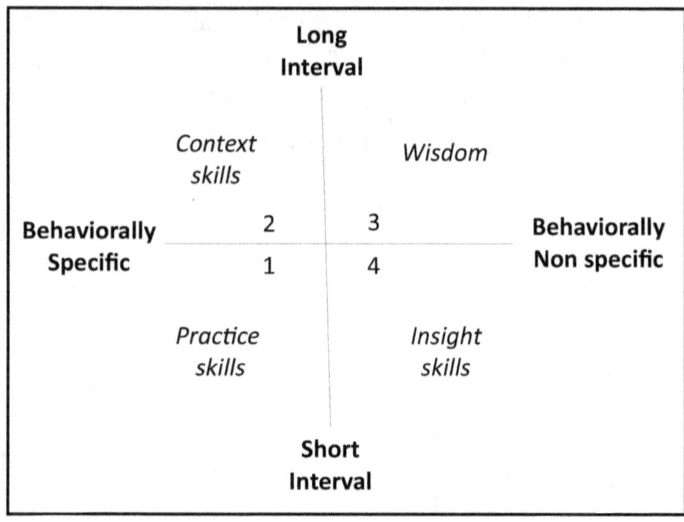

Figure 2 : Managerial Skill framework

Outdoor action learning:

Far from the fanciful images it is sometimes given, outdoor development has real – world focus with a natural skills orientation. Not surprisingly, this is an orientation necessary for managers in the last decades of the last century. As one international observes put it: The contribution of management development that is most important is the pragmatism and people skill its participants develop- mainly through contact with the real world'.

Outdoor Management training gives exposure to action learning, exposure to others from outside cultures, informal shoulder – rubbing, and so on, with the best of management development, in the form of risk tasking, accountability, and access to older, wiser managers who can share their insights about organization.

There is an element of 'action learning' in the model for outdoor development, whereby managers 'learn by doing the thing.'" The principle of action learning were taken up by the EEC's Foundation for Management Development (EFMD) when it stated: 'New approaches in educational technology for large audiences, action research and action learning...... should be broadly experimented with and promoted. These principles can easily be applied to outdoor managerial development. At the heart of action learning is the ability to extract from the new task itself a sustainable desire to known what one is trying to do, what is preventing this and what resources can be found to get it done by overcoming the obstacles. Usually, the process require the help of a small number of people who are also on the same quest.'

Learning by doing:

Professor **Revans** said that it was rather '**learning to learn -by-doing with and from others who are also learning to learn by doing**. The focus is, then, not on the knowledge of the teacher, but rather on the experiences and the needs of the learners.'In Particular, the outdoor development programme emphasizes one of the options of actions learning whereby an **unfamiliar problem is studied in an unfamiliar setting.**

The physical task at the core of outdoor development courses, whether they be abseiling a rock face, climbing a mountain peak or navigating rapids in canoes. Are real tasks, which present real problems to real people in real time with real constrains. Unlike simulations and case studies, the physical tasks are so desired that the manager will experience the practical outcome of his own actions or decision, thereby creating a learning process which could lead him to modify his behavior or options. As such, the physical tasks in the outdoor development courses, dependent as they are on small group work, constitute 'action learning' experiences which stand on their own.

The managers in action courses run by the COSMOS, trust claims to turn out managers who are able to act more positively and flexibly as managers of groups, communication, decision makers and team members'.

John Adair is the founder of **"action – centered leadership,"** which has enjoyed wide application throughout British industry. According to the action – centered leadership model, an efficient manager needs to have:

1. Technical competence to manage the technology of the job;
2. Knowledge of the functional area of management; and
3. A cluster of management skills required to motivate people to work for corporate goals.

Testing Managerial skills:

The skill area is most relevant to outdoor development what, then, are the specific managerial skills, which can be practical and reinforced through outdoor activities? A list of these skills would include:

1. Observing;
2. Selecting pertinent data;
3. Diagnosing problems;
4. Formulating solutions;
5. Deciding;
6. Communicating;
7. Motivating.

Across the spectrum, the physical activities can range from sample rock climbing, where groups achieve goals, to survival exercise, where individuals are left on their own to find routes while living off the land. It is quite obvious that the physical activity must be suited to the desired outcomes.

For example, one of the desired outcomes of the Leadership Trust's management training is to help a manager learn ways of handling and controlling himself effectively even under pressure. The training is reinforced by a tutor attached to every six to ten students who in effect provides a model example of such control in his own behavior. The tutor also holds the safety of the group and establishes the integrity and boundary of the group in which the member can become freer and freer to express himself. The tutor creates a membrane of safety and supports for the group. He makes sure that each person has at least one, usually two, opportunities of leading the group and experiencing support.

Each group, in turn, tests itself out in the three physical activities: sub – aqua diving, rock climbing and canoeing.

The Physical activities themselves comprise only 8 percent of the course content, but they are crucial because they are used to wrench people out of their normal patterns of behavior and mind sets. The physical activity is a powerful vehicle. It is important that it be totally real because then you get real emotion, real fear, high anxiety, high or low morale, real aggression and real learning.

Effective programmes that takes managers out of the classroom and into the outdoors should result in personal development, team development and manage focal points where there is convergence of inputs from management training which include managerial principle and skills, and inputs from the outdoor environment as shown in.

Figure 3

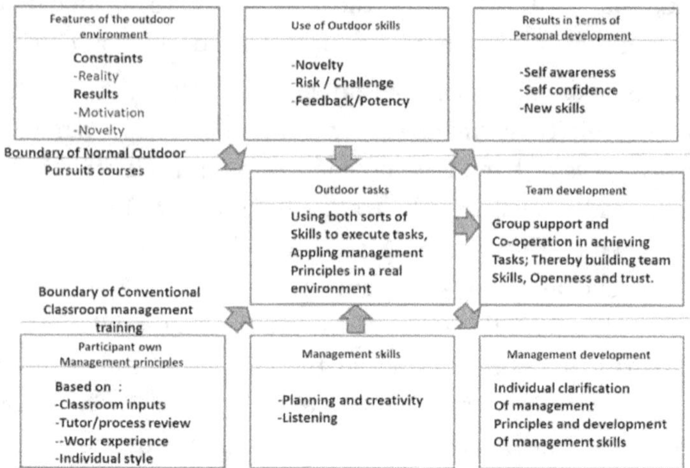

Figure 3 : Linking the environment with management development A basic model

As with physical skills, managerial skills are developed through frequent use and reflective practice. Various participative methods can be used to sharpen diverse managerial skill's. An attempt to illustrate the range of application of participative methods together with their peaks of effectiveness is made in **Figure 4.**

Following this insight, if a company wanted to develop in its managers the skills of observing, it would get best results from field work activities. To develop the ability of its managers to select data, the company would have the most success with the incident method. There would be little point to using the case study method for developing either of these two skills because in that method the observing and data selection are done beforehand by the case writer, not the management student.

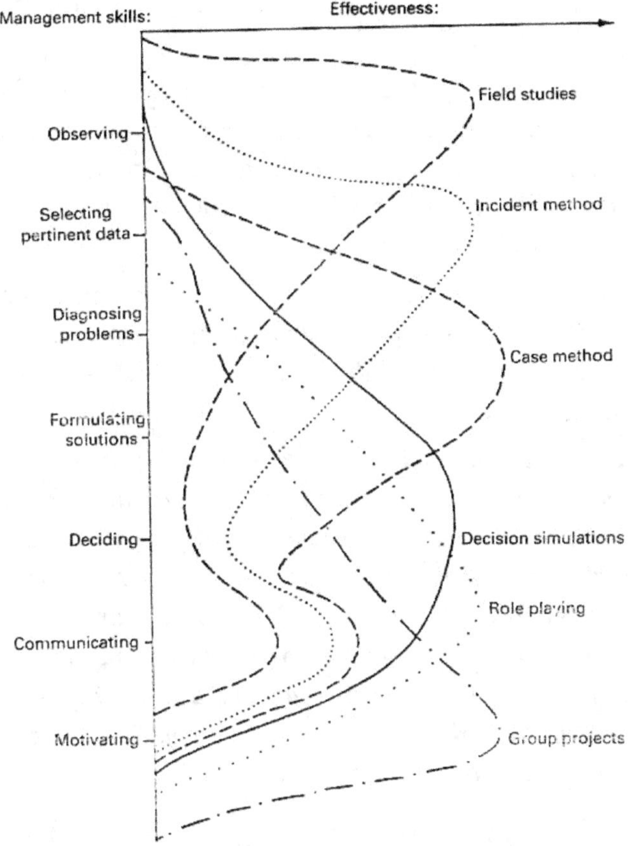

Figure 4 : Effeciveness of participative methods

The strength of the case study lies in its aptness for diagnosing problems and formulating solution. A well written case study is a testing ground for competing managerial judgments on concrete issues. Yet case studies have their drawbacks. 'When it comes to learning how to make sound decisions, the case method is far from how to make sound decisions, the case method is far from ideal because there are no penalties for proposing wrong decision; as there are no real consequences, solutions can be proposed light-heartedly'.

On the contrary, the action – based studies in outdoor development activities are very real and the penalties for wrong decisions are painful; the consequence of bad judgments can be as being lost in a cold rainstorm at the edge of a dark forest.

The food, Drink and Tobacco industry Training Board in its several years' experience with outdoor development training has emphasized the objective of managing change and uncertainty.

"The results of their action are immediately apparent, providing clear evidence of their performance and a basis of feedback, questioning and experiment. Although the outdoor tasks are not normal, they are inescapably real. Managing an outdoor situation is like managing life- it is full of unpredictable events and people, a result has to be achieved and there are only limited resources and time valuable. Because the tasks are so different from the normal work situation. The underlying management processes are laid bare."

Chris, a strong believer in outdoors!

Chris Bonington [The first Mountaineer to climb Everest from difficult South-West face] is a believer in the reality of the outdoors to sharpen managerial action. Executive decision making, participative leadership, team building, the management of uncertainty, motivation, dealing with industrial relations (a threatened strike by the Sherpas while he was on Everest Expedition) are all part of the life and death reality of a major mountain climbing expedition. These aspects of management are as real as the logistics planning and stock control for which Bonington used computer programming. He feels that in climbing Everest in 1975, he encountered nearly 'every type of management problem one could think of. His many Himalayan expeditions, beyond the scope of outdoor development for managers, have all been an extreme confirmation of the power of the outdoors as a vehicle for managing uncertainty.

5. New found confidence!

The use of the outdoors for training by the military goes back to the earliest days of military training. There is no record that Hannibal first trained his troops in the Alps before crossing them. There are hundreds of outward Bound schools in more than 20 countries today and their ongoing influence on outdoor development is considerable. The founder of outward Bound was Kurt Hahn, a German- Jewish educator, who earlier developed the Salem School in Germany in 1920 as an antithesis of the authoritarian German schools of the time.

WOS-B:

We would consider using Outdoor Development if senior management declared a policy of 'True Darwinism' within the organization.

The managers in rough clothing with maps in hand converged on an old trunk half hidden in the middle of the forest. They opened it to find ropes and a pulley and the directive to use the equipment to get the entire team across ravine in two hours. 'This is a "WOS-B"! said to one manager who had been an army officer. The other younger managers did not known what the word meant, nor did they understand the strong emotion behind his statement. They were unaware of the "WOS-B" root of outdoor development.

'WOS-B' stands for **"War Office Selection Board"** which deals with officer promotion in the Army in the first instance and in the second for challenging outdoor problems like the ones used by the war office selection Board for assessment of the men before it. The Navy has a corresponding Board called the Admiralty Interview Board which uses similar group exercise to sort out candidates.

1.   The military;

2.   Outdoor sports;

3.   Outward Bound;

4.   Outdoor education through the school system;

5.   Other youth activities, such as scouts and the Duke of Edinburgh Award, etc and

6.   Organizational development (OD).

The military

The use of the outdoors for training by the military goes back to the earliest days of military training. There is no record that Hannibal first trained his troops in the Alps before crossing them. Today, all branches of the military use the outdoors to train their fighting men, to develop their officers and to select out elite crops.

The selection course for the British Parachute Regiment, for example, which eliminates two – third of all candidates who attempt it, gives the men less than two hours to complete a ten-miles battle march, carrying 13 KG packs, 10 KG of webbing and a 4 KG rifle. After struggling through mud and water and hillsides, the men are kept awake all night digging trenches, doing exercises and fending off instruction who creep up on them and attempt to steal weapons and equipment. At down, the candidates run a six -and –a half mile stretcher race across difficult country in teams of eight, each man carrying 80 KG on his shoulders. They must then go round the assault course three times in under seven and a half minutes and complete the steeplechase within 18 minutes. Finally, they have to carry telegraph poles over rough terrain in less than 15 minutes and do a 14 mile march over harsh Landscape. The Para leadership maintains they are not out to break men but to 'make them, to find the man 'who doesn't quit, who has the robustness of mind to keep going when everyone else falls.

While outdoor development programme have neither the rigor nor the 'selection intent' of such military activities, they do draw on some similar activities, such as an assault course or challenges like crossing a deep chasm with ropes and pulley. Dipping into military handbooks for physical tasks and outdoor exercises which can be used on outdoor development courses is quite legitimate, provided these activities are modified to take account of the age and physical fitness of the managers; and the primacy of learning over the physical task in outdoor development.

Outdoor sports:

Outdoors sports, such as mountaineering, sailing, white water canoeing, caving, diving, orienteering and running, continue to feed the outdoor development movement for managers like underground streams feed a spring. As each of these sports has rewritten with new techniques and equipment, there have been spin-offs for the outdoor development movement. Outdoor development borrows heavily from the sports and is interested in the techniques and equipment and making participation in the outdoor activities safer and more meaningful. Usually, the physical instructors for outdoor development courses are accomplished one or more outdoor sports and this reinforces benefits derived from the sports.

At times, the mere presence of the instructors, fit in mind and body, among a group of over – indulgent, unit managers, generates some soul-searching. Doubters of the ability men and women have regain fitness and a love for physical exercise should examine the phenomenon of running in America. A decade ago only three million Americans engaged in running as a sports and the image of the beer – drinking, TV watching, sedentary American male was widespread. Today, over 30 million American run as sport, many of them participating in demanding marathon running, 42.195 kms.

Not only does outdoor development drawn on outdoor sports for many of its physical activities; the trust of using the outdoors for managers among enthusiasms for outdoor sport can awaken commitment to a lifestyle of more demanding physical exertion.

Outward bound:

There are hundreds of outward Bound schools in more than 20 countries today and their ongoing influence on outdoor development is considerable. The founder of outward Bound was **Kurt Hahn,** a German - Jewish educator, who earlier developed the Salem School in Germany in 1920 as an antithesis of the authoritarian German schools of the time. His opposition to the Nazi regime won him a prison sentence in 1933, but influential friends got him released and out of Germany. He went to Scotland where he founded Gordons to unschool in 1934. His Philosophy of education stressed the development of a student's inner resources as well as intellectual and ocean rescue. At the outbreak of the second World war, Hahn helped to set up a school for British merchant mariners at Aberdovey, Wales, specializing in survival training. The school was named 'Outdoor Bound' and that became the name for the international outward bound movement dedicated to Hahn's Philosophy of education. The Aberdovey school is now one of the leading outward bound School in management education and in the rough economic climate of Britain in the 1980s is still in the survival business.

Outward Bound has always concentrated on courses for youth and has funding from industry for such work. Its involvement in management education, according to lan Fothergill, director of the outward Bound Trust and formerly principal of Outward Bound at Aberdovey, is a long-term commitment. Roger Putnam, principal of the outward Bound School at Eskdale, has carried his commitment to management education far enough to purchase a stone mansion near the school's entrance for the education of managers. Personal fulfillment and character building can only aid the managerial role, 'said a Cranfied, MBA student making the link between the course and his job. But Outward Bound is reaching far beyond its own roots to deal with management development in all its many facets.

The American outward Bound schools have made a good deal of the running with outdoor development in conjunction with business school and universities and at times, private organizations like the center for Creative Leadership.

Outdoor education:

Outdoor development has roots that are seldom acknow-ledged in outdoor education, which is a term now widely accepted as covering educational activities concerned with living, moving and learning out-of-doors. These activities include camping and residential experiences and skills requiring physical endeavour and observation of the environment. Outdoor education, then, is not a subject, but it provides opportunities to complement learning planned by the school. Its goals are to instill respect for oneself through the meeting of challenge and adventure, for others through group experience and shared decision making, and for the natural environment through direct experience.

The focus in outdoor education is on personal development of the young students/learner and the outdoors is seen as a powerful pedagogy for teaching self- reliance, cooperation, confidence, imagination, inventiveness and a capacity for sustained physical Endeavour – all of which virtues are important in the work and in the building of a strong society.

Outdoor education occurs, in one form or another, in most if not all countries of the world. However, it can be implemented very differently, depending on the cultural context. Some countries, for example, view outdoor education as synonymous with environmental education, whilst other countries treat outdoor education and environmental education as distinct. Modern forms of outdoor education are most prevalent in UK, USA, Australia, New Zealand, Europe and to some extent Asia and Africa.

UK

After the Second World War many local authorities in the UK emulated the Outward Bound principles and set up their own outdoor education centers for school children. Visits to these outdoor centers were often subsidized, allowing many children from the towns and cities a unique experience of the outdoor world.

By the late 1980s most UK local education authorities had an outdoor education centre, and there was a growing private sector offering similar experiences. Government moves to offer more autonomy to schools have badly affected this provision. Under regulations for the local management of schools that took effect in England and Wales from 1992 onwards, the majority of the money spent on education in the UK now goes direct to the school, and local authorities often find it difficult to subsidize their outdoor education centers. As a result many have closed.

One of the most significant changes in outdoor education in Great Britain came as a result of the Lyme Bay kayaking tragedy in March, 1993. This tragedy accelerated governmental discussions until, in January 1995, the Activity Centers (Young Persons' Safety) Act 1995 was passed through Parliament in January 1995 and an independent licensing authority, the **Adventure Activities Licensing Authority** (AALA) was formed. Overall, the AALA appears to have succeeded in its mission, but it has also created debate regarding whether it is possible for young people to experience adventure in an 'educational way' within tight regulations. Some people view AALA regulations as tight and thus, restricting their opportunity to provide what they believe to be meaningful outdoor education.

One further area worthy of note is the Campaign for Adventure. This campaign started in 2000 following a one day conference titled "A Question of Balance." Since then the campaign has concentrated on lobbying political individuals and parties to support risk taking and to acknowledge and work against the increasing trends indicated by a "culture of fear." This phrase is the title of Furedi's (1997) book, which is heavily cited in recent UK outdoor education literature. As with most political campaigns it is difficult to assess progress but the work of those involved in the campaign can be followed on line consistent with this position, a recent report from the Office of Standards in Education, which covers England and Wales, concluded that outdoor education is uniquely placed to offer structured opportunities for students to identify hazards, calculate the related risks and decide the significance of a risk in order to determine and implement the precautions necessary to eliminate and minimize risk. Students' involvement in risk management makes them aware of potential harm and contributes towards their being able to take greater responsibility for their own and others' safety. While on the surface it may appear to be consistent with the Campaign for Adventure, however there are some significant inconsistencies here worthy of brief explanation. It appears that the campaign suggested that the very idea of risk taking is to be avoided and the role of outdoor education could be to enable students to assess risk and then 'eliminate or minimize' it. A contrary position is taken by the Campaign for Adventure based on adventure and risk as, at least an educational value, and perhaps even as central to life and a way of being, which is threatened by a culture of fear. The Campaign for Adventure believes that life is best approached with a spirit of adventure and that absolute safety is unachievable.

Recently there has been concern expressed about the decline in the number and quality of school trips in the UK.

In 2005 the Parliamentary select committee on Education published a report on 'Education outside the classroom' which called on the UK government to do more to protect and promote outdoor education. In response the government promised to issue a manifesto for outdoor education, setting out what schools ought to offer their pupils.

North america

The origin of outdoor education in the USA is difficult to pinpoint.North American culture, particularly since European colonization in the 17th century, has embraced a pioneering spirit. This contributed to the extensive development of organized camping programs during the 20th century, Outward Bound programs since the 1960s, as well as many related off-shoot programs including Project Adventure, the National Outdoor Leadership School, the ropes course industry, and many other applications including wilderness orientation programs within colleges and universities and adventure therapy. In the 1970's, the Association for Experiential Education was also formed, along with the Journal of Experiential Education which continues to have a strong focus on adventure education scholarship and practice.

Germany

The term 'outdoor education' doesn't seem to have an exact equivalent in the German language although Kurt Hahn, one of key figures in the development of outdoor education in the twentieth century was German. In general, outdoor or adventure education is not as widespread in Germany as in other developed regions, such as North America, Australia, and the UK. However, a closely related educational approach called experiential education (In German: "Erlebnispädagogik") is commonly applied.

Most organizations and companies offering programs and activities based on experiential education for children and youth also offer similar programs for adults and especially corporate teams which are then mostly referred to as 'outdoor trainings'.

Judging from the kind of outdoor training programs available in an internet search, the main clientele of German outdoor training providers seem to be corporate teams and organizations seeking team building and personal development. There is also a wide range of organizations offering outdoor programs based on experiential education for children, adolescents, families and school classes with or without disabilities. German schools have seemingly started to make increased use of outdoor and experiential possibilities when planning their school trips but the experiential approach is rarely implemented in the normal school system and it is by no means as common for school students to experience outdoor education trips as it is in other countries.

Hostelling international (HI):

The **youth hostel** movement was begun in 1909 when Richard Schirrmann, a German school teacher, and Wilhelm Münker, a conservationist, saw the need for overnight accommodation for school groups wanting to experience the countryside. This Outdoor education started with schools being used during the holidays for overnight stay. The first *Jugendherberge* (youth hostel) opened in Schirrmann's own school, in Altena, Westphalia. In 1912 a permanent hostel in Altena Castle superseded the school-building, and as of

2013 a hostel still stands in the castle grounds. Schirrmann founded the nationwide German Youth Hostel Association in 1919. The movement spread rapidly worldwide, leading to the founding of the International Youth Hostel Federation (IYHF) on 20 October 1932 in Amsterdam by representatives from associations in Switzerland, Czechoslovakia, Germany, Poland, Netherlands, Norway, Denmark, Britain, Ireland, France and Belgium. In 1933 **Richard Schirrmann** became the president, but the Nazi German Government forced him to resign by in 1936. After the World War II he resumed as a President and remains President till his death.

This movement is formerly known as *International Youth Hostel Federation (IYHF)*, which is the federation of more than 70 National Youth Hostel Associations in more than 80 countries, including India, which have over 4,000 affiliated hostels around the world. Hostelling International is a non-governmental, not-for-profit organization working closely with United Nations Educational, Scientific and Cultural Organization [UNESCO] and the World Tourism Organization [UNWTO]. HI has also been identified as the sixth largest provider of travel accommodation in the world.

LEAs:

Between 1907 and 1921, **Local Education Authorities** [LEAs] in Europe were empowered to provide outdoor activities for students through vacation school, vacation classes and school camps. By 1928, fifteen LEAs were running school camps and in 1931 camping. The Norwood Report in 1943 argued that there was moral strength to be derived from involving young people in adventurous land- and water-based open – air tasks.

Outdoor education grew rapidly from 1960 when only a couple of LEAs had residential courses for outdoor activities to 1970 when LEAs ran about 400 residential centers. In addition, schools have acquired hut's. cottages. Disused railway stations, village schools and camps. They have also enlisted 300 field study bases and over 500 outdoor pursuit centers and range of residential accommodation provided by voluntary, private or commercial organization to help achieve the goals of outdoor education. Social development was one of the goals which encompassed relating to their teachers in a more human and approachable manner.

Physical instructors:

The grow thin the use of outdoors for management development parallels this growth in outdoor education. Although the learning in outdoor development for managers is at an adult/organization level, it shares some of the confidence-building and team-work experience used in outdoor education. Regardless of age, the outdoors provides powerful learning to the willing student.

Outdoor development also benefits from a spin-off from the growth in outdoor education which created career structures for men and women who share an equal passion for outdoor pursuits and education. The new breed of physical instructors in school across the country are likely to be people with degree who have come up the educational route. Whereas before, the Outward Bound instructor, for example, might have been a fitter from a car factory who had passion for climbing which eventually took over and led him to full – time position in an outward Bound school. The new outward Bound instructor was likely to have been a teacher specializing in outdoor activities. Some would argue that this was a double – edged change. The educational qualifications may have made the new breed of physical instructions more conversant with the academic question of managers, but it might also have stripped them of invaluable business and industrial experience which would have helped them build bridges back to the work place.

Youth activities

A Number of youth programs, such as the Boys Scouts, Girls Guides, the Duke of Edinburgh's Award scheme the sail training Association the Dartmouth Challenge, operation Raleigh, etc, provide meaningful introductions to learning from the outdoors which young men and women carry with them into the adult world of business and industry. The focus of such Youth activity is often 'character-building, but youths readily cope with the moral expectations, adults place on them and they manage to have memorable experiences despite parental demands. The lasting imprint of these experiences is quite remarkable. Most people remember what they were doing when they learnt that president John Kennedy was assassinated because the shock and drama of the event heightened their memory to create an indelible moment. In a similar manner, the drama of outdoor events, like abseiling a 200 – foot cliff, heighten the moment and makes vivid memories and learning easy to recall.

For managers who as Youths have had memorable outdoor experience, adults development programmers link back to the reservoir of good feelings and powerful remembrances. Outdoor development builds on, but also creates, its own series if vivid, indelible memories.

Organizational development:

The overarching field of social technology, of organization change and development referred to as organizational development (OD) is a significant root of outdoor development for managers. The impact of OD principles and technology on industry and business has fed the growth of outdoor development.

Over the years, industrial psychologists made their most important contribution to the success of business by developing technologies for selecting and training employees. A weakness inherent in selection technologies has been their preoccupation with a criterion of effectiveness which reflects a company's past success rather than its future requirements. A weakness if traditional training methods is their poor results in attempts to alter human behavior. Classic examples are human relations training programmes with a heavy knowledge basis which simply fail to change the behavior of supervisors in any significant way. When major changes of behavior are achieved they often clash head-on with the leadership of organizational climate

These technologies of selection and training have not helped companies meet the demands of the third wave', the micro technology revolution which will require whole industries to make radical changes and initiate massive restructuring.

A further failure of traditional selection and training methods is that their focus on the quality of individuals fails to take into account the fact that organizations are more than the sum total of the individuals who work in them. They are rather complex social systems with intricate inter relations between inputs, processes, internal environment and outputs. To focus simply on the individual through selection and training is to ignore the organization as a total system.

OD then is response to the demands of an organization as a total system. Its techniques to solve organizational problems and to meet organizational needs now comprise an expanding technology for interviewing in changing and developing organizations. OD employees a model of charge based on Kurt Lewin's theory which has a three stage process of:

1. **Unfreezing**: a decrease in the strength of old attitudes values or behaviors resulting from information or experiences which disconfirm one's perception of self, others or events.

2. **Changing**: the development of new attitudes values or behaviors through identification or internalization and

3. **Refreezing**: the stabilization of change ata new equilibrium state through supporting changes in reference groups culture or organization policy and structure.

Each technology used in OD may be evaluated according to its power to effect change at all of its stages.

Into this conceptual framework the varied technologies of OD can be fitted. T groups or sensitivity training is an OD technology which consists of a wide ranging assortment of experience based training. The goals content and training styles of T groups are divergent and so are the outcomes. But the primacy they have given to experiential learning has prepared the ground for the different experience based learning found in outdoor development.

Team development or team building is another commonly used and powerful OD technology which directly relates to outdoor development. The objective of team development is the removal of immediate barriers to group effectiveness and the development of self-sufficiency in managing group process and problems in the future.

Beer distinguishes four separate models for team development.

1. **The goal setting model** where goals influence individual and group behavior;

2. **The interpersonal model** with its underlying assumption that people with interpersonal skills can function better as team. The focus is on shared feelings, mutual supportiveness, non-evaluative communication trust and confidence encouraged risk taking and ultimately higher commitment to group goals;

3. **The role model.** A role is a set of expectations and behaviors associated with a given position in a social system. The elements of this definition.

Include: role expectation – the set of structurally given normative demands and responsibilities associated with a position role concept – the individuals own definition role concept – the individuals own definition of how a person in his position is supposed to think and act; and role performance – the person's actual behavior as it relates to his position.

The managerial grid model. Blake and Mouton have created a team development meeting based on their grid laboratory. In this approach each team spends a week applying the grid framework to an examination of the way it operated. There is a heavy use of instruments before this meeting by individuals. In the end the team tries to reach a consensus on its ideal operations and its actual operating. Needs are identified and plans for both individual and team development are made.

Team building on Outdoors generally has most in common with the goal setting model or the interpersonal model, although the role model and grid model could also be drawn on in team building using the outdoors. Yet team building, vital as it is for managers, is one of a half dozen outdoor development goals.

6. Tackling unforeseen situations!

Given a set of novel, Unforeseen and demanding exercise, the participant will dig deep into own resources to find hidden strengths and uncover weakness. One of the personal objectives is developing a commitment to better physical fitness. There is an underlying belief in the real link between physical fitness and mental alertness, high morale motivation and general effectiveness

Outdoor development courses can be used to achieve the following goals:

1. Self-development through personal audit;

2. An antidote or cure for burn – out;

3. An experience of team building;

4. Attitudinal change in the assessment of self and of others;

5. The development of leadership;

6. A living workshop for communication skills; and

7. An experience of dealing with change and uncertainty.

Self – development

Given a set of novel and demanding exercise, the participant will dig deep into own resources to find hidden strengths and uncover weakness. The aim is to effect a confidence – building experience based on extending oneself. In the dramatic outdoor scene, the course member begins to realize that many of the limitations he feels are artificial and self-imposed. Quite naturally he takes stock of his own level of health and fitness measured against his peers and staff members. It can be a salutary experience for an over indulgent executive to abseil a rock face with an amazingly fit climber or for a timid manager to brave the white water of rapids with a fearless colleague.

In this area of self-development the physical environment is used to stimulate personal risk taking exposure and the exploration of one's own rules habits and constraints. Self – development is seen as the unearthing of personal abilities and capacities which makes the person as manager more autonomous.

One of the personal objectives is developing a commitment to better physical fitness. There is an underlying belief in the real link between physical fitness and mental alertness, high morale motivation and general effectiveness. It is felt that the outdoor experience may prompt a participant to develop a regime of regular exercise which is tailored to his personality, lifestyle, age, current level of fitness and personal motivation. There is a potential payoff for both the person and his company here in all areas of works particularly in stressful and demanding situations.

Although a modern manager may work in high tech office he still lives in a caveman's body. His body simply took millions of years to revolve into a form capable of primitive survival for fighting or for fleeing. It needs vigorous daily exercise. It needs to move out of the danger rhythm it goes into when under threat and to relax in a vegetative rhythm where no adrenalin flows.

The communion with nature stimulated by outdoor development opens up reflections on a deeper interior life. As

Henry David Thoreau put it; **I went into the woods because I wished to live deliberately to confront the essential facts of life and to see if I could not learn what it had to reach and not when I came to die, discover that I had not lived.**

An antidote to burn out

The outdoor development experience can also be an antidote to burn out. Burn out is a state many people find themselves in when they have made intense efforts with few or no visible results. As a consequence they feel angry helpless caged and spent. Managers are subjected to this sense of exhaustion and futility and to a higher level of stress.

There is at present a number of descriptions of burn out. **Maslach** who has produced a burn out inventory, defines burn out as a syndrome of emotional exhaustion depersonalization and lowered productivity.

Freudenberger describes burn out as to deplete one – self; to exhaust one's physical and mental resources to wear oneself out by excessively striving to reach some unrealistic expectation imposed by one's self or by the values of society.

Limiting burn out to professionals **Cherniss** calls it a process in which a previously committed profession disengages from his or her work in response to stress and strain experienced in the job. Behavioral symptoms are encompassed in **Veninga** and **Spradley's** definition of burn out as a debilitating psychology condition brought about by unrelieved work stress which results in

- Depleted energy reserves.
- Lowered resistance to illness.
- Increase dissatisfaction and pessimism.
- Increased absenteeism and inefficiency.

Levinson declares that many contemporary managerial situation provides the perfect breeding ground for cases of burnout. The danger of burn out reaches even the chief executive according to **Ginsberg.**

The crawl or climb to the top has been in a substantial number of cases, so tough, tension filled and debilitating, that once there, the base has been firmly laid for a good case of being burnt out. Also when finally at the top, the pressure to prove to others and one's self that it was indeed worth it and that one is the best man for the office to put one's individual stamp as quickly as possible on the organization; to be strong, dynamic, decisive, innovative and right all serve to produce additional tensions which in time bring on the burn out syndrome...

Even if a solid base for being burnedout were not established in the climb to the top, the normal pressures on the top man, the way we accept decisions to be made the heroic, charismatic styles we accept, and the time/tension demands that organizations place, all mean that the top man may be facing the beginnings or advanced symptoms of being burned out.

Tubesings defines burn out in three powerful words as a **personal energy crisis. Potter** includes this essential aspect of burn out in his description of a burnt out person as one who 'cannot muster enough energy to participate in life', or someone for whom 'the vital driving force has become a whimper'. **Freudenberger** calls burn out a 'depletion of the individuals resources, and attrition of his vitality, energy and ability to function'. The state of the art on burn out is nearly as uncharted as that of outdoor development. Empirical studies are missing in both and assumptions and description hold sway. But a relationship between the two phenomena exists and outdoor development is already being recommended by focused companies to counteract burn out. In real world people do not wait for the social scientists to define neatly and operationalise definitions of burn out and gather data on the phenomenon before trying to deal with it.

Outdoor development training programs with their combination of physical challenge and personal reflection can beapt prescription for coping with stress and burn out. **Freudenberger** recommends that companies deal with these problems by sending mangers to workshops and seminars and other off site physical activities where they have opportunities to release frustrations and renew themselves.

Just as self-development need not be a solitary quest, and can be strengthened by relationships with others, counteracting burn out need not be a solo activity. Here again mutual support established on outdoor development management programs and the sense of community can be beneficial.

Team building

With stunning superiority the Man Diesel team propelled Nikhil and team mate Nikita to finish the task and changed all four tyres on Nikita's car in eight and a half seconds.

Team building has always been an objective of successful organization It is well known that one of the strengths of the Special Air Service Regiment (SAS) is rooted in the way that organization builds its teams carefully maximizing each person's strengths and compensating for his weakness. The technology required to achieve as SAS objective is generally learned after the team has been formed. **In the management**

world technology is learned first. Whether the man who knows the technology and is put in changes will be able to weld a team together is often left to chance. Companies do make appeals to team work. One of the more bizarre examples of team building occurred when the manager of the US based IBM sales unit with 100 people rented a sports stadium in New Jersey for an evening. In front of their spouses and children and some top executives all members of the sales team ran through the players tunnel on to the field as their names were flashed on an electronic scoreboard while the crowd cheered.

The anchor is weighed, the sails unfolded to catch the wind and the vessel sets out to meet the challenges of the open sea. It is outward bound. The success or failure if its voyage rests not only on the skills of the individuals and the crew, but also in their ability to work together as a well-motivated and stable team through routine maneuvers and moments if crisis.

The parallel is then rather simplistically drawn between sailing and business activity.

Such team-work also plays an integral part in the success of the modern business enterprise but is often obscured by the familiarity, pressures and stress of the working environment.

Outward Bound creates the opportunity for individuals to learn to work together as a team and to meet the challenges presented by the outdoors.

What participants learn is more than seamanship, rock climbing or canoeing; they learn that each of these activities is a shared experience which depends on co-operation and the assistance of others for success.

They learn that being part of a team is as demanding as leading it and that individual achievement can be magnified through team-work.

In less dramatic ways, most successful companies devote some time building team working and team maintenance.

It is a great benefit to most firms to have people working in a strongly welded team as a corporate entity rather than simply as a group. Yet managers at all levels can easily feel lost in the organization and isolated from others. Social scientist, **Becker,** who documents the essential dualism of people to want both to be part of a team and to be recognized individually. Outdoor development training focuses on the first need, while companies must tend to both. The leadership Trust, states the ability to build and harness cohesive teams to achieve common objectives.

Most outdoor development programmes aim to make participants aware of the need to understand the forces at work within groups and between groups of people. They try to develop in groups shared goals; the realization that the knowledge and skills of each member are needed to attain its goals; a joint feeling of responsibility for the attainment of goals; and a strong desire to operate as a team.

The outdoor development exercises attempt to clear blockages, physical and mental, to effective team work. Among the common blockages are: the wrong structure, poor training, low motivation, poor controls, inappropriate leadership style, bad planning, unclear goals, and uncertain rewards.

Within the span of a few dates outdoor activities teams can be led through identifiable stages. Stage one might be called the **"me first stage."** In this stage people are rather self-absorbed. They talk together but are filled with their individual concerns andopinions. They know very little about each other's needs, knowledge, skills. There is no common concern for each other and no shared view on what has to be done or how to go about it. What leadership that emerges is often egocentric and fails to assess the abilities within the group. In a mountain rescue exercise forexample a self-appointed leader failed to discover that a member of his group had been in the army medical corp. knew exactly how to treat the injured climber but shyly held back as the group went from one blunder to another.

Another identifiable stage to team development can be called the **"king and his court stage."** A leader takes charge of the group and organizes it under his tight control. He is the focal point of the group and makes the decisions. He distributes parts to others in limited roles he defines for them and coordinates the parts into a whole. For rather straight forward simple tasks this style of team management does work. But the king styled leader cannot handle complicated tasks. He soon suffers from system overload and simply cannot make all the complicated decisions quickly enough. The members of the group – his court – lose energy and the goal often eludes them. The next stage of an effective team is **"the half way there"** stage. During this stage the team starts to get to grips with working together. Interpersonal relationship issues methods of joint working and even the principals of participation come into play.

The final stage is that of a **"fully developed team"** At this stage leadership is determined more by the situation than by the force of a single leader's personality. The role is often shared or rotated to best suit the situation. The fluidity and flexibility of the team's operation is one of its strengths. An open exchange among the members is common as they go to the heart of the issues and deal with substantive matters and problems. A synergy develops within the group as people's abilities and talents combine to give the team a power greater than the sum of its individual parts.

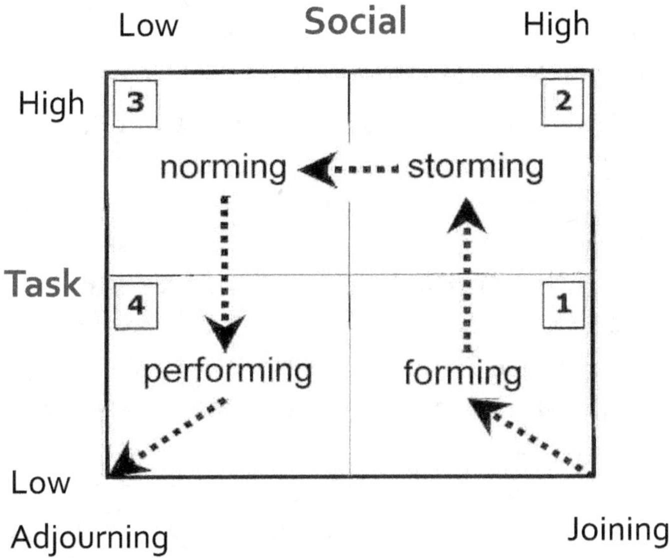

Team building Model

Stage 1: Forming

– The team is created with clear structure, goals, direction and roles.

Stage 2: Storming

– The team refocuses on its goals, breaking larger goals down into smaller, achievable steps.

Stage 3: Norming

– Members shift their energy to the team's goals and increase in productivity.

Stage 4: Performing

– The team makes significant progress.

Stage 5: Termination/Ending

Forming:

Supervisors need to be directive during this phase.

- Team initially concern themselves with orientation accomplished primarily through testing.
- Team members get to know one another, and their respective strengths.
- Team members are focused on themselves and tend to behave independently and to show their best behavior.
- Testing allows to understand how each member of the team works as an individual and how they respond to pressure.
- Testing also allow to establish the dependency relationships with leaders, other group members, or pre-existing norms.
- The team learns about the opportunity and challenges, and then agrees on goals and begins to tackle the tasks.

Storming:

- Team members open up to each other and confront each other's ideas and perspectives.
  - ◉ what problems they are really supposed to solve,
  - ◉ how they will function independently and together, and– what leadership model they will accept

- The maturity of some team members usually determines whether the team will ever move out of this stage.
- This stage can become destructive to the team and will lower motivation if allowed to get out of control.
- Supervisors may still need to be directive in their guidance of decision-making and professional behavior

Norming:

- Team members adjust their behavior to each other as they develop work habits that make teamwork seem more natural and fluid.
- Team members begin to trust each other.
- Motivation increases as the team gets more acquainted with the project.
- Team supervisors tend to be participative more than in the earlier stages.
- Team members can be expected to take more responsibility for making decisions and for their professional behavior.
- Team members work through this stage by agreeing on rules, values, professional behavior, shared methods, and working tools.
- Some members can begin to feel threatened by the amount of responsibility they have been given.
- If the norming behavior becomes too strong, teams may loose creativity.

Performing:

- Teams are now able to function as a unit as they find ways to get the job done smoothly and effectively without inappropriate conflict or the need for external supervision.

- Team members have become interdependent, competent, autonomous and able to handle the decision-making process without supervision.
  - Supervisors of the team during this phase are almost always participative.
- Many teams will go through these cycles many times as they react to changing circumstances.
  - A change in leadership may cause the team to revert to storming as the new people challenge the existing norms of the team.

COSMOSO outward Bound Pioneers enjoy working with managers, tries to archive fifteen qualities with the teams he builds. These are:

1. Good communication within the team and with others outside the team.

2. Active listening where members of the team learn to reality hears what each is saying.

3. Self-knowledge where team members openly recognize their own strengths and weakness.

4. High trust in which the members share a common purpose and trust each other. Energy is spent clarifying facts, deciding on the best methods of solving problems and exploring alternatives. They do not seek to bluff trap or score off each other nor do they distort, withhold, or manipulate information and ideas to suit individual goals.

5. Willingness to use help – a readiness to turn to others both inside and outside the team is developed.

6. Cooperation is the watchword both in joint problem solving and in sharing workloads.

7. Supportive help – an umbrella of supportive relationships is extended over team members sub ordinates and superiors.

8. Collaboration – a spirit of collaboration within the team and with other teams replaces destructive competition.

9. Creative conflict is fostered instead of dysfunctional conflict.

10. Open leadership issues. The pecking order is eliminated from team work; rivalries for leadership diminish as responsibilities are shared and accepted.

11. Meaningful meetings – consensus not compromise prevails in group decision making.

12. Action – things get done there is little waste of energy.

13. Good decision making based on facts not opinions takes place.

14. Goals known and achieved – individuals and the team have the satisfaction of realizing objectives.

15. Reviews of both task and process. The team is interested in what it is accomplishing (task) and also how it is working together (process)

When and Why team members give up?

In a study of 569 managers, they reported that they limited their efforts or input in over 56% of the teams in which they participated. The major causes for giving up were as follows.

- Presence of someone with expertise (73%)
  — **I wasn't needed**

- Presentation of compelling argument (62%)
  — I didn't have other information for an argument
- Lack of confidence in ability to contribute (61%)
  **— I wasn't prepared or there were
  Other "High Power" people.**
- Unimportant or meaningless decision (52%)
  — why waste my time?
- Pressures to conform to team decision (46%)
  — Group think at its best!
- Dysfunctional decision making climate (39%)
  — you want me to risk what?

What to do about team failures?

- Learn about teams. Don't invest in anything without first finding out what it will (or won't) do for you
- Learn before you leap. Visit other companies, read, send people to conferences, etc.
- Develop your vision and strategy. Create a specific picture of what you want to have in place
- Explore readiness. Take a careful look at where to start
- Choose the right team structure to fit your needs
- Craft a plan. You can't implement workplace teams in an ad-hoc fashion
- Focus on real work. Effective work teams get high quality results with high levels of engagement and satisfaction
- Expect transition time. Success won't happen overnight
- Form friendships. A "best friend at work" is one of the most important factors that contribute to high performance teams

- Fire people who refuse to join in

- Give permission to start over

- Appreciate how powerful teams really are. The momentum they bring can be unstoppable and highly influential

Assessment

Assessment is an ethical issue in management education. Business schools, as a policy, do not provide companies with specific feedback on individual management student performance. Such feedback could compromise lecturers and would certainly be regarded as a threat by executive students. By setting to one side such assessment, the business school created a protective environment where the management student feels safe to explore issues, techniques, skills, without the feeling that his company's personnel director is lurking somewhere in the back ground waiting to talk with the lecturers, to take a measure of his performance, to compare him with his peers, to weigh his promotion potential.

This ethic is usually adopted by the organization involved in outdoor development management education, particularly when such activities are joint ventures involving say an Outward Bound School and a university's business studies department size up particular managers, but rather to foster self-assessment and a safe environment in which course members are free to evaluate each other's performance and to offer helpful appraisal of behavior, as two experienced trainers in his field suggest:

"Our objectives for the programme were several fold: For the participants as manager, we would provide a series of opportunities for him to take a complete view of himself as a resource and to extend his capacities to meet a complex variety of managerial situations. We would provide him with opportunities to see himself as others see him and to reflect upon those views, adapting his own behavior if he so chooses."

Whether the course participants are undertaking a management course with an experience based outdoor learning module or are on a contract company course, there is bound to be reassessment of others. The sudden change from the classroom or company offices or factory floor to the rock face or the rapids forces participants to evaluate each other in new role sets with entirely new demands.

The development of leadership:

The latest company based research in America argues convincingly for an exploration of leadership by managers. The chief executives of the most successful US companies require leadership skills – a strong leader (or two) seemed to have had a lot to do with making the company excellent in the first place. The great leaders leave behind a legacy that their successors must protect. The leadership task of the chief executive is to manage the values of the organization. They demand high quality in their product and employed ideas and treat them like adults, allowing talented people long together for experimenting.

All experience – based outdoor training for managers has the development of leadership as one of its objectives. The leadership Trust, for example, in its promotional material sets out its philosophy of leadership, which is quite prescriptive.

Leadership is both a science and an art. The scientific or head aspect refers to its principles, methods and functions. It involves problem solving, establishing objectives, planning, organizing and decision making. The art or heart aspect refers to the intangible human factors. These are personal qualities, personal power, morale, motivation and the vital areas of human relations, such as trust and integrity. Leadership starts with knowing and controlling oneself so that one may approach and handle people and situations right. This means learning to use both one's head and heart positively to win the commitment and involvement of people to achieve a common purpose.

Leadership development therefore begins with defining individual's innate leadership qualities and then enhancing them with the knowledge, skills and self-confidence to be able to apply them effectively. Our course enables people to learn from practical experience which recreates the real and similar problems, pressure and situations that confront us at work. The essential learning comes from the constructive feedback and skilled tuition provided in the reviews after every practical session. The Leadership Trust provides an environment where managers can practice leadership, make errors if necessary, gain constructive feedback and learn without threat to their self-confidence or career.

The objective of giving people the experience of leadership in a practical way where there is minimal risk to those being led is akin to efforts which have been a part of military training for decades. Work in training for leadership, undertaken at the Royal Military Academy and the Royal Air Force demonstrates that to improve the effectiveness in any organization five areas must be carefully studied. **The first**

of these is the structure of the organization which should allow many opportunities for the practice of leadership under varying degrees of supervision. Likewise a tradition of good leadership should be part of the organization's value system. Second formal courses on leadership should be developed to the highest standards. Third such course work should be tied in with subsequent practical leadership training in the officers' training programme. Fourth staff members should be given the opportunity continually to study and improve their performance in leadership training. And fifth a small research and advisory team should be created to maintain and improve standards.

Interestingly outdoor development programs give attention to all of these areas in establishing course objectives and in setting objectives for their own staff development. This is one of several areas for reciprocity between outdoor development organizations and management schools. Business schools use the skills of mountain instructions to create experiential learning for their management students. In return they might offer to the mountain instructors experiences of the business school environment where they may learn more about the theory and practice of management in a classroom situation for their own development and a further enhancement of their dealing with managers on the rock face. In describing its Leadership development programme the Colorado Outward Bound School says the course is offered in the fall and spring with the outdoors as the teaching medium for leadership skills. While the course focuses upon leadership skills taught are applicable to any walk of life.

You will participate in teaching, leading, following project presentation planning and organizing activities. In the end you'll develop the knowledge experience and sense of purpose to act effectively. In addition you'll learn general mountaineering backcountry first aid and emergency procedures how to deal with wilderness hazards, group dynamics and counseling skills. You'll explore the moral, social and spiritual dimension of leadership.

Communication skills workshop

The word communication' comes from three Latin words the preposition *cum* with the word *unus* meaning **one** and a corruption of the verb facere **to make.** Thus the complete word means literally **to make one with.** Not surprisingly, improving communication skills is one of the objectives of most outdoor development training courses.

COSMOS Outward Bound Pioneers uses transactional analysis in their development training. The Leadership trust employs transactional analysis is an aid to self-awareness and self-control for handling and approaching people and situations properly and to develop leadership skills. The Outward Bound course employs a TA consultant who helps design the courses and plays a leading role in debriefing the adventure exercise and group dynamics using transactional analysis.

Dealing with change and uncertainty

The coming shake up in the industrial world due to the widespread use of the microprocessor and the impact of new technology will make the role of the manager more critical. The so called third wave will bring on massive social upheaval as things fall apart and entire new systems of automation and industrial organization emerge. The manager will have to cope with uncertainty and change on a scale which is unprecedented. To carry people along with him during such dislocations will take leadership team work and new ways of coping and prevailing in uncertainty.

Finding new ways to develop an understanding of change and skills for coping with uncertainty seems imperative for educators and trainers of tomorrow's managers:

Much management education has fallen down in failing to relate theory to the hard practical world of managing resources and people and taking the consequences of decisions. No business game, no simulation, no case book study can ever approach the reality because the inevitable emphasis is on the intellectual framework of a problem and not on living inside a word which contains unpredictable personalities and events in which the basis of management may change from minute to minute, and in which the only thing certain is that nothing is certain.

Mangers when placed in the training situation created by an outdoor development program are uneasy about the unfamiliar scene. They are not comfortable with projects on the rock face, the assault course or the canoe route. Decisions are called for in a context of great change and uncertainty and the physical and emotional effects of these decisions are felt immediately and at times painfully.

Managers often deal with problems that are known and methods that are well tried -these present little difficulty. It is when the problems are unknown and the methods are known or the problems are known and the methods are unknown that the difficulties increase.

<u>Nature of Method of Solution</u>

Unknown   Known

2	1
4	3

Known

Unknown

Outdoor development is particularly suited for dealing with box 2 and 4 problems according to Roy C. Williams, head of Training and Development for Imperial Tobacco Ltd. Roy Williams summed up the reasons for using outdoor development: it offers reality (no simulation) consequence (not just theory) direct feedback an opportunity to manage space distance and time and genuine engagement in the tasks (the difference between reading a manual on abseiling and doing it). He said his managers found outdoor development courses vivid and memorable which made the transfer of leaning back to the company easier. He had data to demonstrate the high transference. He also found outdoor development highly flexible in design so that he could use it at one end of his company for the board of directors to develop better strategic planning and at the other end for trainees and apprentices to initiate them into management concepts. Ongoing evaluation of the outdoor programs had made the tailored courses powerful at all levels in the company.

7. Getting the most out of outdoor training

The support of top management is critical for effective outcomes from any training or organizational change effort. Outdoor programmes in particular, run the risk of seeming irrelevant, so it is especially essential that top managers show their support. From practical standpoint, an effective outdoor management training programme requires adequate facilities, trainers and technical and logistical support. Facilities do not have to be remote, but an off – site training location is usually best. In any case programme planner must limit or eliminate trainee interaction with the job environment during the outdoor stage. Most on-site programmes are hindered by inevitable distractions.

Critics charge that outdoor management training is nothing more than an excuse for busy managers to take vacations on company time. But such programmes can be a viable approach for developing management skills, if they are designed and executed according to sound learning principles.

Does such high impact training make any difference in participants attitude and work behavior?

Does it affect organizational outcome?

The issue is open to question!

With many management developments "FADS" – such as sensitivity training or management by objectives – outdoor training may be short lived due to poor application of otherwise good concepts and practices.

So how do you get the most out of outdoor training programme?

What are the essential elements of an effective outdoor training programme?

Sound learning theory:

Outdoor training can easily become a "vacation" or a "fun" break from the routine work. After undergoing unique outdoor activities, they come away with a good feeling and with few new insights and skills. If developing management skills is the goal, then the programme must be based on sound learning theory. The learning model is proposed by D A Whetan and K S Kameron [Refer the chapter Enhance-stimulate –speedup: A case study.: Table 2]

1. **Skill pre-assessment**: Examines participant's current levels of knowledge and skill competence.

2. **Skill learning**: Teaches correct principles and presents the rationale for specific behavioral guidance.

3. **Skill analysis**: Provides examples of appropriate and inappropriate skill performance and analyzes behavioral guidelines and why they work.

4. **Skill practice**: Gives trainees the chance to practice the behavioral guidelines and adapt them to their personal styles, while receiving feed-back and support for trying new behaviors.

5. **Skill application**: Helps transfer learning to real life situations and foster ongoing personal development.

Support:

The support of top management is critical for effective outcomes from any training or organizational change effort. Outdoor programmes in particular, run the risk of seeming irrelevant, so it is especially essentialthat top managers show their support. Unless line staff and human resource staff in the organizational unit participate in this programme together, an outdoor training programme will not work effectively.

Link to strategic goals:

The strategic goals and priorities of the sponsoring organizations should serve as the foundation for the design of an outdoor programme.

You can identify the specific needs through interviews with sponsors, human resource specialists and programme participants. The basic question is what kind of capabilities are needed in the organization to further the strategic goals.

Key question for the design is How does the outdoor training relate to past or current training efforts? What specific skills and concepts are to be developed in the outdoor programme? What is the appropriate format, including programme length, number of participants and levels of participants? What are the criteria for selecting participants? What level of involvement of in-house people and consultants has in the execution?

Once the goals are set, they must be translated in to specific behavioral skill outcomes. Which then serve as a basis for the concepts and activities in the programme.

We use the pre outdoor module of one or two days just prior to the outdoor phase to introduce trainees to the basic conceptual framework. This stage serves several important purposes.

1. It introduces the basic management concepts and skills identified by the needs analysis.

2. It provides a common language and reference point for the outdoor stage of the programme.

3. It begins to establish programme expectations.

The great outdoors:

Following the pre-outdoor module, participants enter the outdoor stage of the programme. It lasts for two or five days. It consists of carefully selected "initiatives."

A central question in planning for this stage is What skills seem most relevant to outdoor training?

Obviously not all training needs can be addressed with this approach. Out door training is an appropriate vehicle for addressing group effectiveness. They are as follows

- Developing self awareness
- Risk taking.
- Communicating support.
- Giving and receiving feedback.
- Problem solving.
- Decision making.
- Assessing and using resources.
- Managing conflict.
- Team building.

Leadership is the composite of various skills of those listed above. These are Some pertinent questions to ask in structuring the programme:

- Are the initiatives arranged in a appropriate sequence?
- Do they lead towards accomplishing the programme objectives?
- Is there any flexibility in the structure of the programme to allow for adjustments in how the initiatives are set up or arranged in sequence?

Skilled Facilitation:

For the trainees to get the most out of the experiences, they need skilled facilitator for those discussions. The key questions are:

- Can programme facilitator anticipate the nature of the information generated and relate to the needs of the participants?
- The processing of the information that emerges from each outdoor initiative is key to the learning process. And participants must also explore their relevance to the work setting.
- What does this experience and the learning derived from it, have to do with the work environment?

In our debriefing period after an outdoor initiative, we usually ask participants to reflect silently and respond in writing to five questions.

- What happened?
- How did you feel about it?
- What principles did you learn?
- How does the learning apply to your situation?
- What do you intend to do about it?
- Trainees write their answers in "learning logs" especially designed for this debriefing.

Transfer of learning skills:

The critical failing of most training programmes is that they lack the means of transferring the training to the job. This is a particular challenge in outdoor training because of the uniqueness of the experience.

First the learning log serves as a means to data collection throughout the outdoor stage of training, facilitator ask participants to identify what they have learned from particular initiative and to relate it to the job environment. Trainees then document specific actions that they can take back to the job based on what they learned.

Each participant is also asked to select a fellow trainee as her or his "coach" during the outdoor phase. Because of this they share their experiences and discuss possible transfer issues. When trainees declare their intentions to each other, they enhance their personal commitments to doing things differently when they return to work.

Another critical activity at the end of this outdoor stage is goal setting and action planning for transferring the training to the job. As raw materials, each trainee uses the learning goals that he or she has written throughout the activities. Participants share their goals and action plans with their coaches before they leave the outdoor environment.

Follow-up and Networking:

About four days after the outdoor stage of the training, participants attend a one-day, post outdoor session. It has several purposes:

- To follow-up on the transfer process.
- To identify and solve the major road blocks to transfer that the trainees may be experiencing.
- To foster networking among participants.

- To get the trainees' feedback on the training, to be used for improving the programme for future participants.

The basic assumption of this stage is trainees were able to develop a supportive climate to practice skills in the outdoor environment, but the work environment is probably not as supportive.

That means that participants must be prepared to create a supportive environment as a means for reinforcing learned skills until those skills become internalized.

Participants are asked to refine their goals for effective transfer and to widen their support systems for reinforcing newly learned skills. In addition, trainees are encouraged to use the network of fellow outdoor training graduates as a source of ongoing reinforcement and support.

The post outdoor session provides an opportunity for participants to relive and refresh their experience.

Skills training and supportive network alone will not result in lasting behavioral and organizational change. Other institutional supports – such as organization's strategy, structure, reward system, and culture – must be consistent with the learned skills. The effects of even the most thorough programmes will be short lived without support and reinforcement for the skills that have been learned in the outdoor programme. Human resource systems of selections, appraisal, compensation and development are particularly relevant to maintaining the desired skills.

Programme evaluation:

Despite the call for more rigorous evaluation of training programmes, relatively few carefully conducted evaluations have been reported.

The sponsoring consultant or organization may not be interested in formal evaluation beyond the traditional "Smile sheet." It may be due to the relatively high cost associated with rigorous evaluation or simply to the lack of evaluation skills among the HR manager.

The difficulty of accurate evaluation deters many organizations from attempting it. It can be very difficult to detect changes in organizational out puts or specific behavioral changes among trainees. Even the most careful study may have trouble isolating the effects of the training.

Despite those limitations, some form of evaluation must be built in to the design of an outdoor training programme. The evaluation can include all the Kirk Patrick's four levels of evaluation criteria: attitudes, leanings, behaviors and outcomes.

Obviously, as one moves from collecting data on training attitudes to examining real, on the job outcomes, the richness of the information increase. Unfortunately so does the cost of evaluation.

Nevertheless, evaluation does several things to enhance the effectiveness of the programme.

- It helps to clarify the purpose and objectives of a programme by forcing the company to be specific about which skills it wants to develop and how those skills will be measured.

- It communicates to sponsors and the participants that the programme is being taken seriously.

- It offers an opportunity for learning and means for refining programme objectives and design for the future.

Sound foundation:

Interest in Outdoor training programme continues to increase, bur the jury is still out on whether they are a fleeting fad or an effective new addition to the management development curriculum. Primary evaluations of programme outcomes are positive, but some practitioners still ignore the conceptual and practical base for effective programme implementation.

Without that sound foundation, outdoor training will not yield positive results. It will likely become just another fad. That would be unfortunate, given the early enthusiasm for what appears to be a high-potential approach to management development.

Facilities and capabilities for Outdoor programmes:

From practical standpoint, an effective outdoor management training programme requires adequate facilities, trainers and technical and logistical support.

Facilities do not have to be remote, but an off site training location is usually best. In any case programme planner must limit or eliminate trainee interaction with the job environment during the outdoor stage. Most on-site programmes are hindered by inevitable distractions.

Facilities need to be elaborate. Many outdoor initiatives can be developed with relatively little cost and it does not work to any level of satisfaction.

8. Enhance – Stimulate – Speedup

A case study

Do outdoor training programmes really work? This research report based on Industries in Aurangabad, sheds light on the topic and offers suggestions about how to integrate outdoor programmes in to their training efforts.

Outdoor Based Experiential Learning Model:

Outdoor environment is increasingly used as a training and development medium for people at various levels. OBET is also known as Outdoor Management Development [OMD] or Adventure Based Counseling [ABC]. This programme comes in two major types. One is low impact programme wherein limited physical risk is involved. Activity involves an entire work group. The other is High impact programme where high physical risk is involved. In our studies, we have used Low impact programme. The foundation of the concept is "Learning through personal experience." It involves series of situations where defined tasks are to be completed, within the given constraints. These constraints are real in terms of time-recourses-people. All these constraints are designed to create pressure under which one has to take decisions and maintain group morale. As the group moves through these exercises, they get the time to reflect on their experience. This facilitates personal learning. They are also helped in relating these earnings to their organizational reality. As a result they come out with these experiences with heightened self-awareness, greatself-confidence, grit to face risk. Though the programme is in open environment, it is not a course of adventure, not a test of physical endurance. It necessarily requires an attitude to enjoy some pleasurable feelings of discomforts. In every situation some adventure is involved. There is an element of risk and unknown which have to be overcome by the physical and mental skills of an individual. Here meaningful challenges were presented within the framework of safety. This programme was implemented during August 2009 to April 2010, in five companies in Aurangabad city. The programme schedule was as per the **Table 1.** We followed the D A Whetten and K S Cameron learning model. This model explains the relationship between learning in five stages. The learning model is as per the **Table 2.**

With this fact in view we implemented a model of "Outdoor Based Experiential Training Programme" [OBET] to catalyze the process of learning in five industries in Aurangabad city, Maharashtra state, India. 1. Expert Global Solutions Pvt. Ltd. 2. Man Diesel 3. Sanjeev Auto 4. S S Controls 5. Aurangabad Electricals."**COSMOS Outward Bound Pioneers, India** "[Outdoor Management Development consultant] conducted OBET programme in an open environment of Patnadevi Reserve Forest, near Chalisgaon, Maharashtra and Hiranya resort, Foot hills of Daulatabad fort, Maharashtra.

All employees were trained from the above mentioned 5 different organizations.Evaluation methodologies used in this research were as follows.

1. Participant's responses on questionnaires filled out both before and after the OBET programme. For which we used D A Garvin evaluation system.We evaluated

four attitudes from this system **a.** Systematic problem solving **b.** Experimentation **c.** Learning from experience **d.** Transferring knowledge.

2. Supervisory reports on the functioning of the work group before and after an OBET programme.

3. Interviews with managers to get their reactions to individual and work group performance after an OBET programme.

The initial goal of our evaluation efforts was to determine what behavioral changes, if any occurred after people participated in OBET. We evaluated two types of behavior by applying **Kirk Patrick's Model.**

1. Individual behavior. It includes **a.** Locus of control **b.** self-esteem **c.** Confidence in peers **d.** Faith in peers.

2. In Group behavior we evaluated **a.** problem solving ability **b.** group cohesiveness **c.** Group clarity **d.** Group homogeneity **e.** Group effectiveness.

D A Garvin system:

Questionnaire analysis for dynamic learning by D.A. Garvin evaluation system shows that in all the four areas a. Systematic problem solving b. Experimentation c. Learning from experience d. Transferring knowledge. there is a significant rise as per **Table 3.**

Effect on individual and group behaviors

The participant self-reports we gathered have consistently have shown a significant improvement in the overall functioning of a work group after a group attended an OBET programme. On the other hand, no significant change have been reported in Individual behavior after the programme. The results are shown graphically in **Graph 1.**

The participants:

The evaluation results described above strongly suggest that low impact OBET programmes are effective in improving group process and interaction skills. But the improvement did not occur uniformly for all participants.

In the programmes we studied, we looked at several participant variables that could influence OBET effectiveness.

1. Whether a programme was conducted with intact or non-intact work group.
2. Whether participation was voluntary or mandatory.
3. Gender composition of the group
4. Whether the group supervisor was present for the programme.

We will look each of the four variables separately.

1. Intact or non-intact work groups:

Some team building programmes train workers who are strangers to each other at the start of the training. Some organizers believe that strangers often react more honestly with each other than do people who work together every day.

Our results show that intact work teams [those who interact at work on a regular basis] benefit significantly more by attending OBET programme than do people from non-intact work groups.

2. Volunteers or non-volunteers:

Most of the training manuals suggest that only volunteers should attend training programmes. Our observation and evaluation suggest that it is not true for OBET.

Despite having been forced to attend the programme, the non volunteers' behavioral changes were not significantly different from those of the participants who volunteered to attend the programme.

3.   Gender composition:

We ran all three types of programmes from all males to all females. Most groups attending OBET include both men and women.

Our observation shows that a statically significant relationship between the balance of Men and women in a group. Changes in two key areas like problem solving and overall group effectiveness showed more improvement than did groups that were male dominated or female dominated. The group with a balance of men and women also reported that they enjoyed the OBET programme more.

4.   Presence of supervisor:

90 % of the groups we evaluated attended the programme with their supervisors.

We expected the presence or absence of supervisors to have an influence on the effectiveness of the programs. The only significant effect the supervisor's presence had was that the group that attended OBET with their supervisors liked the programme better. As far as changes in group behaviors, we found no significant differences attributable to the presence of the supervisors.

The training programme:

The selection of activities indoor or outdoor was made by the individual facilitators and varied from programme to programme and from group to group. We were able to evaluate two variables in the programme.

- The amount of training held outdoors.
- The use of follow up programmes.

The first of the OBET variables is the percentage of time spent outdoors. It varied from 80 percent to 50 percent. The average amount of time spent outdoors was 65 percent.

Many people argue that the outdoor settings enhance the success of this type of training. Our observation does not support that assumption. The amount of time spent outdoors during the training programme was looked at was unrelated to the success of the programmes.

It will be interesting to compare those results with the programmes that are held entirely outdoors or indoors. Our observation strongly suggests that the process not the settings, facilitates the behavior changes.

We studied the use of follow-up programmes three weeks after an initial OBET session. Transfer of training normally declines after a session is over. So most trainers recommend follow-up sessions to reinforce the original training.

The different programmes had three follow-up conditions

- No follow-up.
- One hour general discussion programme three weeks after the training.
- One-and-a-half-hour session using experiential activities, three weeks after the initial programme.

We found no significant difference in participant's behavior among the three groups.

Ten Recommendations:

The following 10 recommendations grow out of our research They may help the organizations using the OBET.

1. Determine the objectives of the programme before you select the type of training to use. Decide the focus first, Team building or Leadership, communication etc.

2. Use OBET only if it appears that this kind of training will meet your objectives. Low impact OBET programmes seem most effective in such areas as problem solving and team building. Other types of OBET programmes may be more effective in developing other skills.

3. Select a consulting and training firm carefully. Decide whether the firm's role will be to design and facilitate the entire programme or to train your in-house facilitators. Pay attention to educational background and experience. Most consultants in this new field have recreation and counseling degrees but little business experience.

4. Train – the – trainer sequences should pay particular attention to human behavior skills and organizational knowledge.

5. Focus your low-impact OBET programmes on intact work groups.

6. Let the supervisor of the group decide whether to attend.

7. If possible mix men and women evenly in the OBET programme.

8. If an outdoor setting is not feasible, use experiential activities as a part of your outdoor training programme.

9. Focus on the Quality of the initial OBET training. But be sure to design appropriate follow-up option.

10. Evaluate the effectiveness of your OBET programme. Maximize the results by modifying the programme based on evaluation.

Table-1. OBET Programme Schedule.						
Stage	Month	Expert Global Solution	Man Diesel	Sanjeev Auto	S S Controls	Aurangabad Electricals
I. Needs Analysis	August 2009	Visit to all the five companies				
II. Pre-Outdoor	September 2009	Slide shows on "Concept of OBET" in all the five industries				
III. Outdoor Activity		a+b+c	a+b+c	a+b+c	a+b+c	a+b+c
	October 2009 Batch I	10+25+5	10+25+5	10+25+5	10+25+5	10+25+5
	November 2009 Batch II	10+25+5	10+25+5	10+25+5	10+25+5	10+25+5
	December 2009 Batch I	10+25+5	10+25+5	10+25+5	10+25+5	10+25+5
	January 2010 Batch II	10+25+5	10+25+5	10+25+5	10+25+5	10+25+5
	February 2010 Batch I+II	20+50+10	20+50+10	20+50+10	20+50+10	20+50+10
IV Post Outdoor Session	March 2010	Visit to all five industries. Feedback meeting with the staff.				
V Programme Evaluation	April 2010	Meeting with the staff and presenting the report.				
Key: a: Sr. Managers, b: Engineers c: Supervisors						

Table 2
DA Whetten and K S Cameron Learning Model.

Relationship between Learning Model and five stages
Emphasis given in stages.

Sr.No	Elements of learning Skills	Stage I Needs Analysis	Stage II Pre-Outdoor	Stage III Outdoor Activities	Stage IV Post-Outdoor	Stage V Programme Evaluation
		Company visits	Introduction to OBET through indoor slideshows	Patnadevi Reserve Forest	Follow-up	Kirk Patrick's Evaluation
1.	Pre-assessment	2	2	0	0	0
2.	Learning	0	2	1	1	0
3.	Analyzing	0	2	2	1	0
4.	Practice	0	1	2	1	0
5.	Application	0	1	2	2	2
Key:- 2: Major Emphasis, 1: Minor Emphasis, 0: No Emphasis						

Table 3

Questionnaire analysis for dynamic learning by D.A.Garvin evaluation system.

Attitudes	Expert Global Solutions			Man Diesel			Sanjeev Auto			S S Controls			Aurangabad Electricals.		
	Score			Score			Score			Score			Score		
	B	A	R	B	A	R	B	A	R	B	A	R	B	A	R
Systematic Problem Solving	12	15	3	11	13	2	15	32	17	15	30	15	12	18	6
Experimentation	13	15	2	11	11	0	17	25	8	11	16	5	13	16	3
Learning from past experience	11	13	2	11	11	0	25	32	7	17	25	8	12	17	5
Transferring knowledge	11	13	2	11	12	1	16	22	6	11	18	7	13	15	2

Key:- 1. B: Before OBET, A: After OBET, R: Rise in the score.

2. Minimum score=11 : Environment not conducive for dynamic learning.

3. Maximum score= 44 : Environment greatly supports dynamic learning.

Kirkpatrick's Evaluation Model

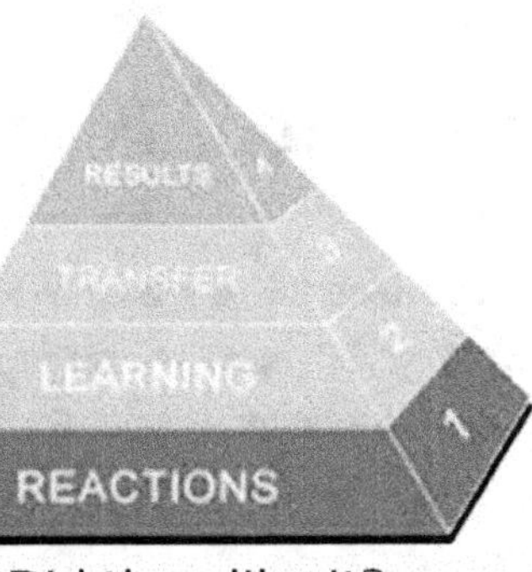

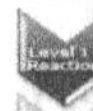

- Did they like it?
- Did they learn it?
- Did they use it?
- Did it impact the bottom line?
- What is the Return on Investment?

Group behavior before and after OBET by Kirk Petrik's evaluation system

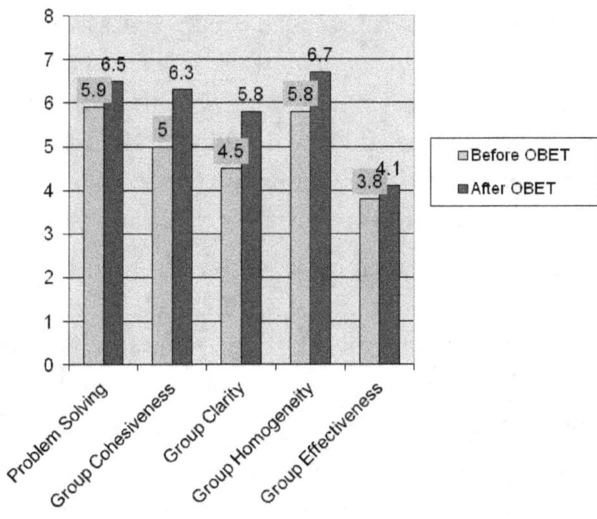

9. Revolution or Fad?

Outdoor Training promises to be a major HRM trend from 1990s. More and more organizations are investigating outdoor training programmes for individual managers, management teams and work groups. However on the other hand some say that "Outdoor programming is nothing more than an opportunity for organizations to pack whole management teams off to risk life."

More and more organizations are investigating outdoor training programmes for individual managers, management teams and work groups.

More than 200 training organizations currently offer some type of Outdoor training, also known as adventure or experiential learning. Such programmes are designed to develop leadership and teamwork skills through structured outdoor activities. There are many Multinational companies who have developed their own outdoor training programmes. Many universities are sending people "into the wood." as a part of their traditional executive education programme.

But is outdoor training a revolution or a fad? At one time or another, American organizations have tried virtually everything in pursuit of more effective managers and teams.The most intriguing aspect of the outdoor training movement is the intensity of the debate regarding its usefulness as a training strategy.

Even the top executives are among the converts. Nelson Farris, V P of Nike Corporation says "I think every one of our employees should go through outdoor programmes, not just some people." He says "We are looking for ways to get people to open their minds and deal with the process of change. This programme will help our company."

But outdoor training has also evoked opposition. Skeptics content that such programmes are a waste of time and at worst harmful to managerial effectiveness.

More than three decades ago Ron Zemke suggested "Outdoor programming is nothing more than an opportunity for organizations to pack whole management teams off to risk life and limb together" Jack Falvey argued in the Wall street Journal that "building outdoor party games and simulations, when the real work is to be done is all around, should be grounded for managerial malpractice indictments."

Despite all the controversy about outdoor training and despite the dramatic growth in corporate spending on such programmes – many management and training professionals have little understanding of what outdoor training is, where it came from or what it aims to do. Most managers have heard or seen something about "This outdoor training stuff" but want to reserve judgment until they learn more about it.

Handfuls of training organizations are using outdoor training from the last 20 years. There was no organization in the world using this outdoor training concept before 1980s. In fact most outdoor programmes were created only during last 10 years.

Two kinds of programmes:

Outdoor training reflects the images like rafting down the white water. For others it meant taking "Trust falls" from

5 feet platform. Others thought it meant participating in group problem solving and team building exercises etc. All are right. These different images reflect different levels of outdoor training activities.

Current practice can be categorized in to two major types.

1. Wilderness Programmes.

2. "Outdoor centered" programmes.

In **wilderness** programmes participants live outdoors and engage in strenuous activities such as mountain climbing activity or white water rafting or sailing etc.

In **outdoor centered** training there are two kinds of rope courses.

1. ***"High ropes"*** activities take place well above the ground.

2. ***"Low ropes"*** courses rarely get higher than eye level. They can be "team courses" that focus on "problem solving" or "individual initiative courses" that focus on individual problem solving.

Training centers offer different mixes of High Rope and Low ropes training in their programmes.

Some of the controversy over outdoor training stems from confusion over the different types of training available. For example, arguments about safety are more applicable to wilderness and high ropes experiences than to low ropes courses, due to the greater likelihood of serious accidents. Confusing the different types obscures the potential benefits and liabilities without increasing our understanding of outdoor training.

Wilderness programmes attract Top executives, Middle level managers, low level supervisors and even non managerial workers. Group that work together in office often participates together in the programmes and such approach gives favorable results.

"A Typical programme":

In a typical programme a facilitator – generally responsible for 8 to 12 participants – begins by discussing individual and group goals for the programme. An individual goal might be something like, "I need to work on my listening skills." A group on the other hand, may be trying to enhance its understanding of the group process. Then the participants are gradually introduced to the experiential training process, their unusual learning environment and their fellow team members. It starts with simple activities like basic worm up and then proceeds further.

Issues and concerns

As with any type of training programme, the success or failure of outdoor training can be determined only if the purpose of the programme is known. Unfortunately, most outdoor training programmes apparently do not start with any clear objective. This suggests that outdoor training is often initiated with little planning. Perhaps in an effort to accomplish something for which it is not well suited. More than 70% of the organizations do not evaluate their Outdoor training programmes in any way.

Training organizations also need to evolve more systematic evaluation methods so as to determine the effectiveness of outdoor training for developing skills useful in the corporate context.

One detailed study was reported by Christopher Ronald in an unpublished doctoral dissertation, "The transfer of outdoor managerial to the workplace." Ronald study looked in to middle level managers who participated in outdoor training. The managers said that, after the outdoor training, they managed their time better and interacted more effectively with their subordinates and superiors than they had before taking the course. Their subordinates and superiors agreed with those assessments.

Other factor that influence the effectiveness of outdoor training:

1. Composition of trainee group [Sex, Age and Educational background]
2. Presence or absence of group supervisor.
3. Whether the group normally works together?

If outdoor training is to be refined and applied where it has the best chance for success, more needs to be known about those group dynamics.

One misconception about outdoor training is that the training will take care of itself. Once the course is designed and exercises are explained. But the facilitator does make a difference. As with any training, the need to train trainers is critical to the success of an outdoor programme. The role of a facilitator is critical and often ignored key to long term success.

It is true that High rope programmes and wilderness programmes can involve high degree of physical activity; they often contain elements of danger to participants.

But it is inappropriate to condemn all outdoor training programmes as physically hazardous. Low rope programmes, common in outdoor-centered training programmes, are less dangerous than high rope courses and some wilderness programmes. Participants in the more strenuous programmes must be carefully selected based on physical ability to participate.

Programmes involving a high level of physical activity are obviously inappropriate for those who have disabilities such as heart problem, high blood pressure. In this situation rather that eliminating the outdoor programme entirely, companies can create alternative training for people who are physically unable to participate in a particular type of training programme.

Some training professionals have suggested that low ropes programmes need not be held outdoors at all. One recent development in this type of programme is "Portable site," which can be carried from location to location and set up in a relatively short time. Such equipment would greatly reduce the cost of developing a site specifically for the outdoor training.

Outdoor training is more than a fad! When all the evidence is in, it will probably rank as an effective human resource development strategy, particularly for enhancing team building for work groups.

10. That is not TARZEN!

When our OMD programme started, Nikhil, operations manager, Human resources asked "Why do we have to go to the woods? Is there any need for such a very different style of management training?" The other Operations manager describes his positive experience "It does allow you to see and learn things about yourself."

It was a group of Operations managers. I use to call them the Tarzens of their company. Nishad says "Those of us who got our OMD training done are currently in assigned leadership role. We are accustomed to performing that role. In OMD we were put in a totally different environment. We do not have a office with our name on our door or an organization chart giving us authority. We have to get out with the peers and work to make the things happen as a team. We have to organize what role each of us can play best to help the team achieve the goal."

"The uniqueness of the environment gave us a chance to look back and see what leadership is all about. Some of us have difficulty stepping out of that take-charge role and stepping in to another very meaningful role. In certain circumstances, in certain tasks you need to be the influencer without being the person in charge." While the outdoor portions of the courses that the participants love and work outdoors, It is not a survival course and not be confused with such programmes as Outward Bounds.

"People have fear of the outdoor, that they will be uncomfortable. The fact is that the restroom facility may be less than wonderful, but the food is good, and nothing they are asked to do is physically stressful."

The outdoor is an effective way to look at leadership. On the job technical expertise masks leadership capabilities. Knowledge is not leadership. But the outdoors strips an away subject matter expertise. None of the tasks we ask these people to do are anything they have any idea how to do, in most cases. All that is left to the leader is his or her ability to co-ordinate the ideas and abilities of the team to get the task accomplished. The leader's role is to provide a central clearing house to get the job done and to empower the team. We think this leadership style more closely resembles the style of the future, when the leader will not be likely to have all the answers.

It gives you immediate feedback on whether you succeed or fall. You know when something does not work. We build a chance of failure in to the exercises with the idea that if the participants experience failure, they will learn useful things. In other words, we create relatively straight forward goals that require a leader to accomplish. These exercises can be debriefed to identify failure.

You need to do a good job Communicating, Listening, encouraging ideas and standing back far enough from the action to have a clear perspective on task accomplishment, team building and individual empowerment to be successful at these exercises. When you fail to do these things, usually the exercise fails. Despite their lack of innate expertise, the managers are given a leadership "model" to use in the exercise. The theoretical model gives them some guidance as well as a framework for performing together. It recognizes the need for a leader to stand back and focus more on the team and the individual to get the tasks done.

The outdoor programme is handled by professional outdoor consultant and emphasizes safety. The indoor programme is designed by consultant. The corporate values are the guiding force behind the indoor exercise.

John Clindenin, chairman of Outdoor company came to the conclusion that the future was going to be very difficult from the past, and how we would respond would depend on our people. That future would require different skills from the past. Outdoor training shall help executives to deal with the challenges of the future.

11. Metaphoric learning: Hierarchy to cluster

True training, in our staff's experience, is about reflecting on and changing people's attitude and/or behavior in a mutually agreed way. OMD programmes should be designed to be fun, engaging & enjoyable, non-machismo & non-threatening and there should be no "hidden agendas."

Mr Kapoor, CEO of the company was looking for a way to create excitement around new ideas. He used the outdoor activities to break through old patterns of behavior. He and his mangers at one point presented to others in his unit a skit in which he dramatized both the old managerial system and the new. His purpose was to develop a small core group of committed people, who could then serve as leaven in the organization in order to achieve change. He could achieve this by making his managers to tackle "Unforeseen Adventure Situations." Participants were given seven unforeseen Adventure situations to be tackled in groups.

Over the rivers and through the woods:

It was a group of 40 key managers and professionals from all divisions of this company. This programme is different from any that this group has been through. The company president is wearing a red T-shirt and the genes. The director of marketing did not shave this morning. The chief financial officer has traded in her high heeled pumps for Reeboks. There is no briefcase in sight.

It is there first adventure learning programme, and despite the preparation session they have all been through, you were not sure what to expect.

The four day programme concentrated on team building and communication. It is not that the team assembled here had anyserious problems, on the contrary you consider yourself to be very pretty effective. But the competition in the business is becoming cutthroat and technology is racing way ahead of you.

As a training professional we spearheaded the movement for some intense team building, to help the company tighten its hold on its slot as a major player in the industry.

Adventure learning or experiential learning programmes use many kinds of challenging outdoor activities – often involving physical risk – to help corporate participants achieve their goals. The goals tend to fall in to two categories.

- Group focused objectives include better communication, more creative problem solving, more effective teamwork and improved leadership. A classic activity for working on group related objective is "The wall" 12 to 14 feet structure that team must get over by working together. The wall can be a metaphor for any business challenge.

- Personal growth objectives encompasses self-esteem, risk taking skills, self-awareness and stress management. "Rope work" like river crossing, rappelling down the rock etc. are favorites for addressing personal growth.

Adventure or experiential learning is a much more powerful way for people to learn, than many traditional classroom programmes. "Learning by doing" is the secret.

A lot of traditional training programmes – many computer courses – emphasize learning by doing. What makes adventure learning courses different is that the learning – and the doing – takes place on three levels, **Physical, Intellectual and Emotional.**

We had a team of 15 managers and they were asked to traverse a swamp. It is marshy area where people do not fall in to. The group members need to get from one side to the other. They may have to bring along a big water drum, planks and rope and blocks. There is no correct way to cross the swamp. A group may decide to create an overhanging rope structure, or to lay out the boards and blocks in a partial bridge and make the trip in stages. Sometime the activity is timed.

This event can teach participants a lot of different things. It is about group dynamics, how the people work as a team, whether they use resources effectively, whether they respect individuals and how they communicate. It may show them whether they are being creative, whether they are listening to, respecting and building on ideas and whether they are focusing on the task on hand.

The lessons vary depending on the work team objectives. We try to spend time upfront with clients to find out what their issues are and to design activities to work on those issues. For example, a group may need to focus on handling conflict within the work team, or building creativity.

If the team is not working effectively at work, it comes out right away in experiential activities. By the end of series of challenges team members have created a clear picture of their patterns as a group. Functional problems at work – such as spending too much time planning or failing to listen to everyone's ideas – become apparent after a few experiential learning events. Adventure learning programmes is a way to enhance, stimulate and speed up the process of organizational change and team building.

Once I had a group at MIDC Lonavala doing a sailing programme. "One guy was steering, and the boat was going back and forth. Everyone else was just sitting around, talking, and not paying attention to where they were headed. They were all trusting the leader and for a long time no one noticed that they had not gone anywhere." Then a person realized that they had passed the same anchored boat floating there as a marker again and again.

When I went for a feedback session, they were doing the same thing in the work place. The work group was going around in circle. Later on I realized that they had fallen in into that pattern. Same register, same agenda, same members, discussing on the same issues again and again, signing the minutes and not arriving to any conclusion resulting in to no decision.

One of the most impotent results of outdoors is a **new found confidence**. "I came out of the programme feeling as if I could do anything" is a common response. This experience injects a shot of self – esteem into everybody so they can take the next step and learn from it. The atmosphere at experiential learning programme is supportive. Team members and counselors applaud each other's efforts and lend moral and physical support throughout the activities. The emphasis is on testing your limits or working together, not on winning a competition.

Trust is a big part of adventure and experiential learning experience. In a **Trust walk** one person leads a blindfold teammate over a course or through the woods, is popular. Many programmes use **Trust fall**, in which people fall backward off a 5 to 6 feet wall, trusting their teammates to catch them.

For some participants the greatest challenge comes from opening themselves to others. Physical risk is just one part of the experience. The largest and for some people, much more difficult challenge is the personal risk of becoming close to trusting other people. Some of these exercises will push hard at people's personal safety boundaries.

For a lot of people, opening themselves to others is the most difficult challenge, the most difficult risk. That is a big part of why we do the outdoor events., to set the stage for that one moment in a person's life when he or she can speak about who he or she is, and be listened to. That is a powerful experience and the outdoor events can really set it up.

A lot of people think that experiential training is going to work magic. It does do a lot of good things, but is only a component in finding out how to meet companies' need. Our approach looks at the self, the work team and the company. We believe that high performing business and teams start with high performing individuals. What makes high performing individuals is taking care of the mental, physical and emotional sides of ourselves... We incorporate fitness of body and mind, as well as the emotional and social side. It makes for a dramatic opportunity for people to take the step, to move forward in their lives.

We can train them towards team work, honesty and empowerment, but they end up as nothing more than buzzwords if we are not constantly making ourselves aware of our self and our teams, of how we communicate and perform. Everyone who works with us gets passionate about our approach because we live the lifestyle we preach.

We are creating not just incremental change, but transformation- in people, and therefore in organizations we do what appears to be adventure training but we do not consider ourselves an adventure training company. It works so well because we add other elements.

Learning the outdoors:

Know before you swing in to action? Here is some advice on what to consider before you take the plunge.

- **Know what you are after**: Have a clear understanding of specifically what your company is trying to accomplish. The more focused you are on your needs, the more helpful a consultant can be in meeting those needs. We do not want to fit square developmental issues in to a round hole. If you know what your needs are, you can fill those needs and you can get your money's worth... Be very clear about the outcome you want, rather than the kind of training you want.

- **Make sure**: that the company you select can tailor its programme to your organization. Pay special attention to the pre-adventure exercises and post adventure follow-up. Ask yourself if the programme is flexible enough on the front and back ends to point back to your company's specific needs. Make sure you use adventure training to serve your purpose, rather than just sending your people to go through a company's programme.

- **Try a test run**: Have a few people from your company go through a programme first. That will help them understand what is possible.

- **Take a careful look**: Ask yourself who is going to deliver the training? Are you believable? Are they just mountain climber or do they have a broader understanding of group dynamics? A lot of companies are very good at doing safe, good experiential learning programme, but are not management and organizational development consultants. They may be able to help you discover a lot about yourselves, but they should be able to transfer it back to the structure and culture of the organization. Unless that structure evolves with the management teams newfound insights, then real change can take place.

- **Send intact work team**: Team should not be disparate to go through the programme.

Some situations are as follows:

Support each other [River crossing]

Trust others [Fall of trust]

"Pamper pole" Reach-stretch yourself [Jump and catch the trapeze]

It is harder to Lead than to follow [Seeing leads blind]

Mistakes are okay [Get across the rug]

Pull together

Rely on the team

1. Support each other [River crossing]:

Santosh Patil stood at the edge of a cliff staring into the emptiness below. A slender cable stretched from his perch

100 feet above the river to a goalpost on the flat ground 200 meter away. He was strapped securely into the harness that was to carry him along the cable and across the river. He was doing it for the first time. It was an unforeseen situation for him. In this he knew there was no danger. But still he had to jump off the cliff. and fall for a while before the cable snapped up his harness and throw him down the line to the landing beyond.

"Go on Santosh, you can do it" several employees called out

Each of them was going to make the same jump. Across the river at the goalpost he could see the group of his friends who had preceded him on the cable. They were also encouraging him to come on. Santosh hesitated only a moment and then gritting his teeth, hurled himself over a cliff in to the open air. He was jerked upright as the cable tightened. Now he was speeding down the cable, the wind blowing past his face, river and the ground beyond rushing towards him. Suddenly he was sliding into the goal. The cable ended and he hung suspended above the ground, swinging in his harness. He knew he had to have support to do it. "I could never have jumped, without those other friends and teachers standing with me on the cliff and encouraging me. "He felt a surge of gratitude and warmth for his friends. "With people like this" he thought "we can accomplish great things both here and back at the business"

2. Trust others [Fall of trust]:

What was Mr Anil Joshi, Principal of Arya Chanakya College doing on the wall about 6 feet above the ground? Managing a residential school with confidence and discipline was looking uncertain and concerned!

Behind his back and below him were five teachers and five support staff of his college.

Some were smiling and some were serious. Mr Joshi seemed uncertain about what was about to happen. He had been told to let himself fall backward off the wall. If all went well, he would be caught by the people standing behind him.

But would they catch him? If the people step aside or let their hands slip off, he would be crashing to the ground.

It was not an ordinary occurrence for a person to fall off a wall. Still he had to try to show courage. After all he was a leader. Some teachers thought the Principal would not dare to fall., that he will find some excuse to step down from the wall. Other group of teachers thought, Mr Joshi has a sufficient courage to fall but wonder whether their colleagues would bother to catch him.

Finally Mr Joshi, steeling himself against his fear, leaned backward and fell suddenly off the wall. Bellow him ten pairs of hands went up and caught him as he fell, and gently lowered him to his feet. Mr Joshi smiles with gratitude. He said "If I could trust you to catch me when I fell, then I must trust you to run the college in my absence, shouldn't I?

"Yes"one answered, and all cheered.

3. "Pamper pole." Reach-stretch yourself [Jump and catch the rope]

Manali Kulkarni, a senior executive from one company looked at a slender pole rising 20 feet above the ground. At its top was a small circular platform just big enough for her two feet. From a nearby tree, a trapeze bar was hanging.

"Just climb the pole" said a supervisor.

She looked with a doubtful expression at a person.

"It is no problem!" he insisted. "There are rings all the way up the pole." "What am I supposed to do up there?" she asked.

"I will go up the tree, and swing the trapeze out to you, you reach out, grab it and swing down" supervisor answered.

"Oh!" Manali said, not at all reassured.

"It is all right" supervisor insisted."I will climb the pole after you and put you in a harness, even you fall off the pole, you won't go very far... and there is a net here too." He said pointing to a light netting that was spread beneath the pole about 5 feet above the ground. "If you feel, the net will catch you, there is really no danger at all."

And so with trembling, sweating hands, Manali pulled herself slowly up the pole, on to the platform at the top.

From across the clearing she heard her supervisor's voice "Here is the bar, I am going to swing it over to you from the tree, you reach out and grab it."

Manali saw the bar coming and began to reach for it. Suddenly the whole pole moved. Frightened, she froze. The trapeze, however had peaked in its flight and returned to the tree. Manali missed the bar twice. But slowly she was recognizing what she had to do. She pushed off the pole with both feet and stretching her arms grabbed for the trapeze.

Now she was no longer on the platform. Instead she is falling through open air reaching madly for the trapeze. She swung with the bar towards safe landing at a shelf built onto the tree.

Caution had discouraged her from reaching for a bar.

"Do not leave your perch," "Do not take the risk," "Stay where there is something solid beneath you."

But she had overcome the pleas of caution, she had abandoned her place of safety and she own the prize.

"I had to stretch myself to reach to do it" she told herself.

4. It is harder to lead than to follow [Seeing leads blind]

The seeing was to lead the blind. Man Diesel company group was divided in to two. Half the group had been blindfolded. The whole group assembled in pairs. One person blindfolded and one seeing. They were in the rock, gravel, steep gullies. There was danger all about for anyone who made a misstep.

It was a simple exercise. Those who could see were to lead those who could not on a half hour walk through a rough country. Each pair of participants was to work out a set of signals, without talking to one another, by which they would progress. Blindfolded person simply place a hand on the seeing person's shoulder and follow in his or her steps. Each pair took off on the course in the rough country. At the finish line, those who had been blindfolded were relaxed. It had been a slow and Pleasant walk. But those who had been able to see were hot, sweating and Uncomfortable. What made them this way?

Nikhil Agrawal says "I was worried that the person behind me would fall and get heart.

"I had to make sure I did not go too fast for her" said Anita Deshpande. "I had to be sure she could follow easily" "You know", said Company CEO Anand Karve removing his blindfold.

"I never before realized how much easier it is to follow than to lead. The follower just relaxes and lets the leader take the responsibility for where the two are going. The leader has to worry all the time about whether the follower is going all right. I had always thought the opposite."

Laxman Mahajan, a smart Engineer says "If the leader wants to delegate to the follower so that the follower can make his or her own way, the leader has to make sure that the follower has eyes to see ahead, like enough information to the subordinates to decide what ought to be done next.

5. Mistakes are okay [Get across the rug]

Two rugs had been placed on the conference room floor. Underneath each was a simple electronic grid. In front of each rug a team of participants from Experts Global solutions Pvt. Ltd. was standing. Each team was to find its way across the rug through a sort of maze created by a concealed grid. The exercise was nonverbal. Words could not be used as a means of communication. One person at a time entered the maze from each team and as he or she took steps on the rug, a buzzer would go off, when the feet were on the wrong path. The purpose of the game was to get across the rug before other team without setting off a buzzer. Initially members of each team picked up his or her way across the rug. When the buzzer sets off, the next person took over trying carefully to remember the false step the previous person had made. Each person was trying carefully to plot his or her own path through the entire maze. Fearful of making an error and setting off the buzzer. Each person proceeded with great care. It was a slow process. Suddenly a person on one team had an idea. Rather than only one person on the rug at a time, several went on, each following directly in the footsteps of the person ahead. Now there was no need of caution. When the leading person sets of the buzzer,the one just behind simply stepped the other way. Now there was no need for delay. As soon as the person buzzed out, another was there to go ahead. Quickly the team made its way across the rug and claimed the victory.

Is there a lesson here?

Could it be that mistakes are okay, as long as others learn from and act on them? Could it be that rather than living in fear of consequences of an error, time could be spent in team work, where error becomes an education?

Yes! Risk taking is necessary to innovation, creativity and successful change. But risk taking involves the chance of error. Dynamic institutions learn to profit from errors, a weak one tries at all cost to avoid them.

6. Pull together

Five teams stood at the ends of five ropes radiating from the center like spokes from a wheel. Each team is engaged in a tug of war with the others over a "pot of gold" situated in the center of the circle formed by five ropes. The winning team would be the one that pulled the pot of gold from the circle in its direction. Once the pot shifted slightly towards one team, but the others redoubled their efforts and the pot returned to the center. They struggled on and on, wearing themselves out but not budging the pot more than a little bit. Finally all gave up in frustration.

The lesson is clear: when people pull against one another, nothing happens. If they want to win they have to pull together.

7. Rely on the team

"I was amazed the first time I saw a wall" Sandeep said.

It was 12 feet high and 25 feet long. They told me I was going to go straight over it., but I did not believe them. The wall was made of smooth boards, freshly painted, and here was a wide dusty open area in front of it. I had no ladder, no stone, nothing to stand on. I reached up the wall and tried to find a handhold., but there was nothing on which I would get a grip. I decided I could not get over it, and I told them so. So they told me I could have a team of people to help me. I wanted rope or steps; instead they gave me several people. And then they told me that we have to get everyone over the wall, not just me.

There we stood in front of the wall. Everyone looked at the wall, then at each other. How to get over? We were given three minutes to talk, plan and create a strategy, and afterwards only to cheer one another on.

We decided we had no choice but to do it by hand. We were going to push someone up to the top, and then he would have to reach down and pull another up, until we had every one over the wall.

One of the men in our group was big and heavy – probably 100 KG when we looked at him, we knew no one was going to be able to pull him up over the wall. Because we would have to push him, he had to be the first one up.

After lots of hesitation, we all took up positions in a little huddle at the base of the wall. Then a big man started to climb up our back. We built a human pyramid steeper and slowly push him up to where, by standing on our back, he was higher than the wall and could throw a leg over to get into a sitting position.

It was easy to push several other people up and over the wall, with most of us pushing from below and him pulling from the top. Then we began to run out the people. For the last two people, we had to build a human chain from the top of the wall down because the big man on the top was not strong enough to pull two up at one time. So we had all those bodies hanging down from the top to get enough arms to pull the last two people up.

We got everyone over, and what an excitement there was then. We felt that we have done a magnificent thing. We learnt that by relying on team we could do what none of us could even begin to do alone.

While going through the above experiences the participants face the real situations which require a group to act as a team, a leader for a particular task to use a whole range of management skills to get the task done. They were required to analyze the information, convince, research, motivate, encourage, support, consult, make judgment, take decisions, communicate, delegate, plan, monitor, control, report, use resources effectively, lead a team, respond to change. All these essential skills for the dynamic learning were evaluated before and after OBET by our supervisor Mr Kishor Bhonsale.

The above exercises are not business itself, of course. They are metaphors for business. Experiential learning is a metaphoric learning, and it will not transfer without careful attention to the process of transfer. This is crucial point.

Experiential learning is marvelous catalyst for changing the attitudes and behavior of people in the workplace, but it is only a catalyst. It can only be used successfully when the ingredients are there to permit the desired reactions to occur in the office itself. Because Mr Kapoor recognized this fact and used experiential learning to help make the transition to the cluster organization, he derived benefit from the investment his company made in extra business activities. Without the structural changes that the clusters embodied the people in, the unit would have been unable to apply much of their learning and the experiential learning would have been wasted.

The opportunity for people

Above mentioned are the powerful lessons for a group of people who are trying to run a business. Instead of supporting one another, many people try to climb to their own success over the fallen bodies of their comrades. Instead of taking risks, many people try to avoid mistake at all costs, fearing that any error will cost them dearly in promotions, pay increases, or even employment itself. Instead of working with others, many people wages a continual battle among departments. Instead of reaching for success, many attempt to do as little as possible always protecting themselves from any risk of failure. Many people spend their energy thinking how much better things would be if they ran the business rather than its executives – forgetting that it is much easier to follow than to lead. Finally many people shy away from challenges not realizing the potential for success that is created when individuals work as a group.

Often a business finds it is in trouble because of these kinds of attitudes and behavior. When the business is having difficulties and those in it want to do things differently take more risks and be more aggressive the lessons just discussed are exactly what people need.

But lessons learned in catalyst exercise, no matter how pertinent, may not transfer directly to business. People may recognize the importance of trust but be unable to trust others in the work environment. They may see how important teamwork can be but be unwilling to give that much of themselves at the office. Or they may recognize the importance of all these lessons, and want to apply them at work, but be unable to do so.

Why might people who want to behave differently at work not be able to do so? First, the desire may be only shallow. After all the work place is far different from a conference center or an exercise field. Different incentives apply. The desire to overcome a challenge in the exercise environment may not carry over into the office.

Second other people at the office may not have been through the same exercise or may not have absorbed the same lesson, and so they find the new attitude and behavior of those who have strange. Those who are not part of the new attitudes may actively obstruct the efforts of those who are. They may be suspicious of the transformation some have gone through or threatened by it.

Finally the circumstances of the office may inhibit the extension of the new lessons. People who want to work as team may not encounter one another. People who feel they should take risks may find themselves in a performance appraisal system that penalized failure, without making allowances for the risks involved and the potential that had existed.

In general transferring the lessons of exercise to business can be very difficult. As a result it is often useful to think of a form of half-life for an attitude change. Every four weeks half the new spirit gained in the exercise is lost until after a few months virtually all is gone.

Moreover things may be worse than before the effort to change. Matter may have deteriorated as result of the process. People who have experienced the lessons and then been unable to apply them successfully at work may be frustrated and resentful. "What has happened to the spirit of the conference center?" they ask each other with anger.

RADICAL TRANSFORMATION: Hierarchy to Cluster

Establishing clusters requires a change process. Change is made difficult by inertia by fear of the unknown by attempts to protect established positions of privilege and by lack of knowledge of how to behave in the new situation. Hence it is not enough simply to have a plan for a transition to clusters. The process of getting there also requires considerable attention.

In general people advance two sorts of objections to a radical transformation. First they may say "We're already doing that. We've been more open in our decision making we're delegating more to people and we're delivering. There's nothing more to do."

But this repose is like that of a person who has a lot of weight and insists on wearing his or her old, ill-fitting clothing. There is much more to do before the full advantages of the organization of the future are realized.

Another objection is that in a cluster no one is in charge. A group without an internal hierarchy speaks to some off anarchy. It is like a scout troop without a leader.

"We're from too many different backgrounds," it is often argued, and too many varying clusters. We have to have someone in charge.

These are powerful objections, less significant in logic than in the emotional commitment to the status quo that so often accompanies them. Logic alone cannot carry a radical transformation. Persuasion on the right side of the brain is also required.

Catalyst help break resistance to change and they help create an environment in which change can occur.

What do catalysts accomplish?

- They provide a forum in which opposing views can be put on the table so that their change process is in the open rather than concealed and undermined.

- They provide a mechanism for letting go. This is most important because many people hold tenaciously to illusion of command and control.

- They begin to build a basis of trust among people in which there can be honest communication. Most people can't work together as teams because of suppressed resentments that have their foundation in past misunderstandings or unsolved conflicts. Unless these barriers can be overcome, there can't really be cooperation. Honest communications among people are less important when people worked on their own, but in the cluster format communication are crucial.

How do Catalysts Work?

In reality, of course, managers in a hierarchy can influence behavior of employees only to a limited degree. Often, little can be achieved beyond minimal performance by hierarchical and directive approaches. Nonetheless, many managers believe that without control the business would sleep their fingers into chaos. And some employees find comfort in the thought that someone else is in charge.

Hence, letting go of the notion of control is a prerequisite to experimenting with clusters. This key to empowerment liberates employees to go beyond what they are told to do and it frees mangers to do more important things than closely supervise others.

Catalysts help people to let go of the old order and to understand that the new cannot be built without relinquishing the old.

Catalysts work by...!

- Creating an environment in which change can take place by making it okay to question how things are customarily being done.

- Building a climate of encouragement and support so that teamwork – which is key to clusters – can develop.

- Providing an opportunity to experiment with trust and self-disclosureina group.

- Being a forum for personal growth and change in which individuals can try out new attitudes and practice new behaviors.

- Allowing opportunities to learn from others.

- Taking the change process out of the solely analytic, rational, and linear and permitting instead a left – brain approach.

Simply thinking about moving to clusters is not enough to help attitudes and behavior change. So an effective catalyst involves emotions and lets people feel what the changes mean. This is a crucial element in the radical transformation of a company.

Alternative Catalysts

Physical activities are not the only type of catalyst, but they are important. Their method is to put people in situations that minimize positional power such as that encountered in hierarchies, In such exercises people can actually watch leadership rotate from those with titles to others who are more competent at the assigned tasks, For example, it is rarely the boss who comes up with the solution for how to get a group of people over the wall.

Further, physical activities put people in touch with fear and, when it is overcome, help to make it easier to overcome the fear associated with a new organization at work. Learning from the activities facilitates understanding in how to let go of control and to work in a freer organization.

In addition to physical activities, there are simulations and classroom type exercises. To many people, simulations are less threatening than physical activities and often have a broader scope of acceptance. Also simulations are less language dependent and are therefore especially valuable with groups of many nationalities.

Case studies, such as those included in this book, help by showing what others have done and how they have solved problems.

Bonding exercises use self-disclosure to bring more of the whole person to the work group, thereby building trust.

Visioning exercises, which I will describe shortly, go beyond the purely rational but without the sometimes perceived limitations of physical activities.

These various alternative catalysts stress different forms of communication. If the medium is the message, employing only words to help people understand clusters is to suggest that the process can occur only in one's head. To go beyond words, facilitators can turn to videos (including those of physical exercises to let people see themselves), music, skits, and so forth.

But is it Brainwashing?

Many types of learning are offered to companies with the ostensible purpose of serving as catalysts to improve the attitudes and behavior of employees. Some are much more extreme than others Many described in this chapter are relatively conservative, derived from military survival exercises, and stress the emotional uplift that comes from overcoming fears in oneself. Other processes involve substantial philosophical and even religious elements.

Most physical activities utilize several powerful psychological tools to assist in breaking through to a new set of attitudes for participants. Among these tools are

- Disorientation taking people away from familiar surroundings and supports (including family and for executives, their secretaries and other staff)

- Egalitarianism removing the comfortable lifestyle many people now have and replacing it with more Spartan circumstances in which people are grouped together and suffer minor deprivations.

- Heavy workload (i.e. lots of planned activities).

- High emotional intensity.

- Pressure, especially from peers, on the individual to perform.

- Unfamiliar challenges.

Emotional tension and pressure are necessary to get people to give the exercises a chance. If people were simply asked, "Do you want to go out in the woods and jump off cliffs?" or "Wouldn't you like to stand on a 20 foot pole and grab a trapeze?" many would say no.

Time and again I have watched people come to the end of these programs with a conviction that they have really gained something significant, However, there is also resistance to such learning. There are stories that in some business programs people have been injured. In some other programmes people have lost their lives (though I know of no specific cases). There are also tales of brainwashing and of exercises that violate some persons' moral convictions. Clearly objections are primarily to physical activities and less so or not at all to simulations and case studies.

Most companies that sponsor metaphoric learning say they do not require their employees to attend. But participants say there is tremendous pressure to participate. If employees refuse, they may be left out of something that is important to the business and their careers may be adversely affected. If people attend the program, they may often find themselves under great pressure from others to participate in whatever occurs. Thus they may be carried along by hierarchical or peer pressure, only to regret it later.

One of the reasons for resistance to these programs is that they have been confused with encounter groups, which have developed a bad reputation. Encounter groups generally operate from the presumption that a better bond can be created among individuals only by first having them be honest with each other about their feelings, including those that are negative. In effect relationship are first broken down so that they may later be built up.

I have heard managers vigorously condemn these sorts of programs. "We just went through a program like that [i.e. encounter groups], one told me: and now half of us hate the other half." Another added "I don't think I 'will ever get some people in my unit to work together again."

Although encounter groups are sometimes used as catalysts in business transformations, many physical learning exercises are quite different. Experiential learning is positive from the start. People are confronted with physical challenges but are encouraged to believe that they can overcome them and when they do, are praised for it. There is none of the negativism that initially accompanies an encounter group approach.

Strategic Visioning as a Catalyst

Experiential activities are not the only catalysts available to organizations that are attempting to develop new attitudes better suited to cluster organizations. An effective alternative has been developed that utilizes a visioning process supplemented by visual representations. Visioning may be used in conjunction with experiential learning of course but there are those who prefer visioning as alternative.

Visioning is a more powerful process, one consultant told me, and you don't have to jump off cliffs.

As practiced at the Pecos learning Center, the essence of the visioning process is to help people think about their business in a new way. From the new modes of thought come ideas about how to serve customers better how to cut costs and, and how to organize and work together more effectively.

What's a car? This is the kind of question with which a facilitator might start a process for a group from an automobile company.

"It's a method of transportation" someone in the company might answer.

What else/the facilitator ask. How does the customer see it?

"It's a lifestyle" offers another "And there are many types of lifestyles each of which needs different kinds of vehicle."

"It is a form self-expression" adds another "The car a person drives is a personal statement about the kind of person she or he is."

The group explores the concepts of lifestyle and self-expression as they apply to automobiles. What would it mean to how cars are designed, marketed, serviced? Insights develop.

Then the facilitator asks for yet another shift in how the group is thinking. This time ideas that appeal to the group are slower in coming, but finally a member observes,

You know, if you think about how cars are used in our cities at rush hours, you get a different picture. They're in the middle of traffic jams. In the summer it's hot outside, noisy, smelly from exhaust fumes. Drivers are frustrated and angry at traffic jam. They're yelling and making obscene gestures toward each other. In that setting the car is not so much a form of self-expression as it is a refuge. It's an island of contentment in a world of confusion. It's my own space where I can be myself and get away from all the bums outside. In Summer it's air – conditioned and cool. In winter it's heated and warm. Its seats are comfortable and just fit me. The steering wheel is right where it suits me. The radio or tape deck plays the music I like. It's my place of escape from the hassles of the world. It's my sanctuary.

"That's really good," the facilitator says. Encouraging others to pick up on the idea, she asks them to think through its implications. How should the company design a sanctuary? How market it?

Ideas pour out and are captured on flip charts or writing boards. The implications of novel ways of thinking about the product emerge. Slowly a plan takes forms-often one that is radically different from the company's present mode of operation.

"Now what will keep us from getting to our new vision of the company?"

Answers pour from the group: This procedure and that structure but also more than procedures and structures, for behind them lie the thought processes that put them there. Can we change the way we think?

"What do we have to do to let to go of ourselves? "the facilitator asks. As insights come from the group, everything seems clear. People are swept up in exhilaration at the freedom that lies before them. Everything seems possible at this moment.

"But what about tomorrow morning?" queries the facilitator, "Will the high last? Will it seem as clear and attainable then as it does now? Will we retain the vision?"

The group has to capture its vision; First, they put it into words. "We need a statement of what we want to be," the facilitator says. "It's got to be short and clear, and no jargon. It's not to be a page from the company's strategic loan. It should stress fundamentals. If we do these things right, then we'll be a business success."

Around and around go the thoughts. Short sentences are amended and become longer sentences. When they become too long, they are junked and the group starts a new.

"We want our vision to coincide with what the customer wants" suggests one group member. "The customer wants something that's not a hassle to obtain and that's fun to have."

"Easy to purchase and a joy to have," proposes another group member.

"You know" adds another, "of we really did that – made it easy for the customer to buy our product and made sure it was a joy for him or her to own – than we'd be a success."

"Only if we kept our costs in line, said another."

"That's right. There are lots of things that have to be done to make a business a success," commented the facilitator. "But keeping the customer first is probably number one. So we've made a good start. What else belongs?"

So it goes an interactive, imaginative group process in which people grasp new ways of thinking about their business and their own role in it.

A vision statement is now on paper. Can it be rendered into graphic form? That is the specialty of a few talented artists who listen carefully to such discussion and portray them visually in full color. When converted to posters and circulated in the office, these pictures remind people of their vision and help keep it foremost in their minds even during the distractions of the day to day business environment.

Changing a Culture

The vision is complete. New attitudes and behaviors are promised by each members of the group to their coworkers. But not everyone in the company has been in the process.

Can the culture of the whole company be changed? What are the catalysts to bring that about? Will it not be much harder actually to implement a new vision that it was to develop it?

Probably it will. An executive of a major pharmaceutical company told me.

We had demoralization and absenteeism in one of our departments. We got the key people together and worked out a new vision of what the department ought to be. Than we began to try to implement it.

We proceeded to hire people very carefully. We screened them for work attitudes and previous behavior as well as work skills. We selected only those with outstanding dependability. On average in their previous jobs, they had attendance records far superior to those in the department they were joining.

After six months we checked the attendance records of the department and the new people. We expected to find a marked improvement in the department's average absenteeism. But we were shocked to find no improvement at all. Worse, the new people we had so carefully screened before hiring. Showed attendance records no better than that of the department as a whole.

Rather than the new people improving the department, the department had worsened the new people. The new People hadn't changed the department. The new ones had been changed by the people already there. The new people conformed to their environments.

I've never seen so strong a demonstration of the power of an established culture in an organization.

In an exactly similar way a few people coming back to an established organization with a vision and new attitudes are caught up in the old ways. And new people brought in from the outside are captured by the natives.

The traditional pattern of attitudes and behaviors in a human organization such as a business is a powerful force, Trying to get people to adapt to a new pattern, such as that which clusters require, is not at all easy. This is why many companies use catalysts such as those I have described in this chapter.

A firm can move to clusters through a communication effort only (i.e. telling people what is coming) but it can get there more quickly and securely with a program that serves as a catalyst to get supporting attitudes and behaviors in place quickly.

Using a catalyst to smooth the transition to cluster organization can be helpful in overcoming the old system. But it is best if the catalyst is not so extreme in its philosophy that it alienates people. Also while participation should be voluntary, it can nevertheless be encouraged. The important thing is to try to get a proper balance.

Australian Walk:
Team work , Communication, Co-ordination and Control.

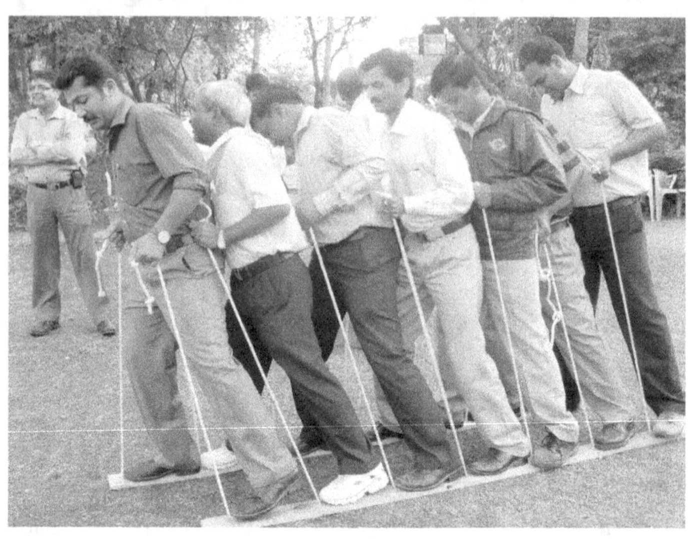

Balloon walk:
Team work , Communication, Being together and Control.

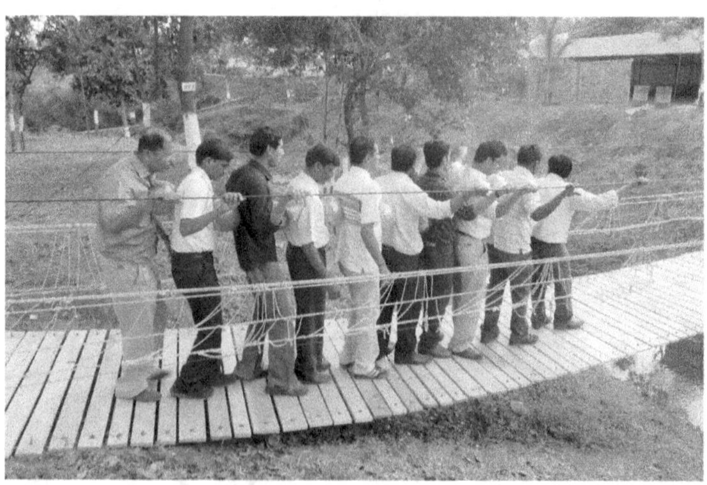

Fall of Trust:
Team work, Trust building, Make judgment, Confidence building, and take decision.

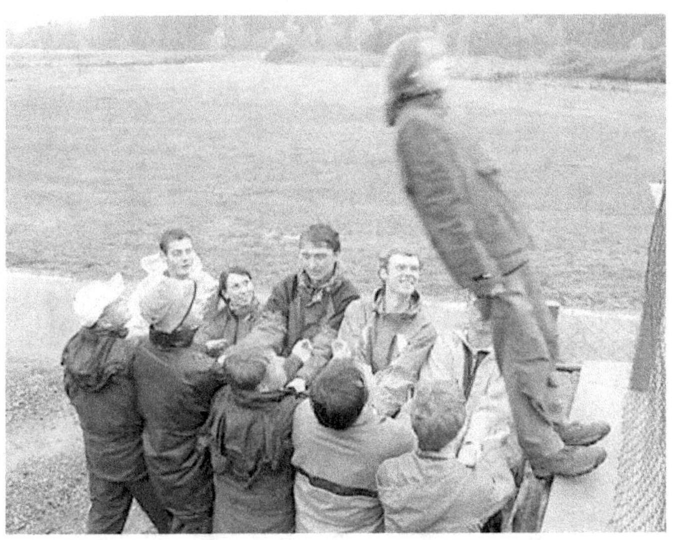

Passing the ring through the body:
Team work, cooperation, planning and carefully examining.

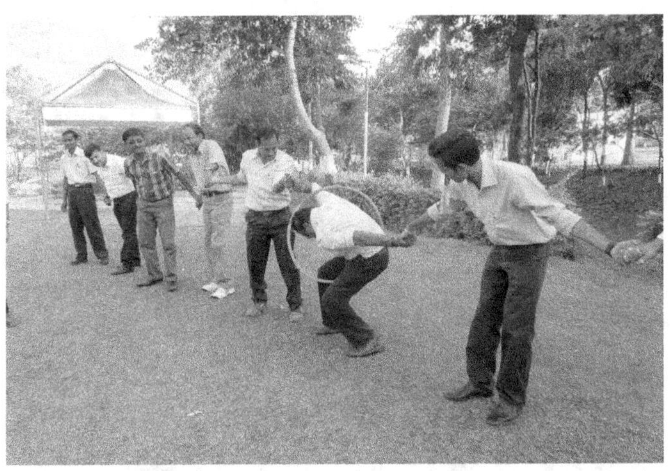

Passing through the web:
Team work, Carefully examining, Communication, support and Strategic planning.

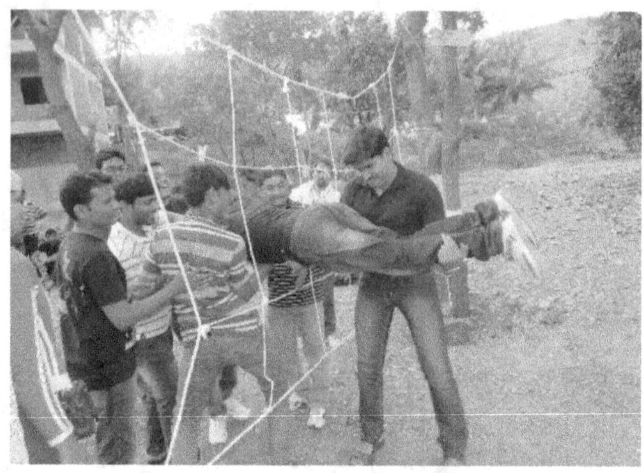

Putting tyre in the pole:
Team work, Identifying core competencies, Resource management, Control, consult, Motivate, encourage and support.

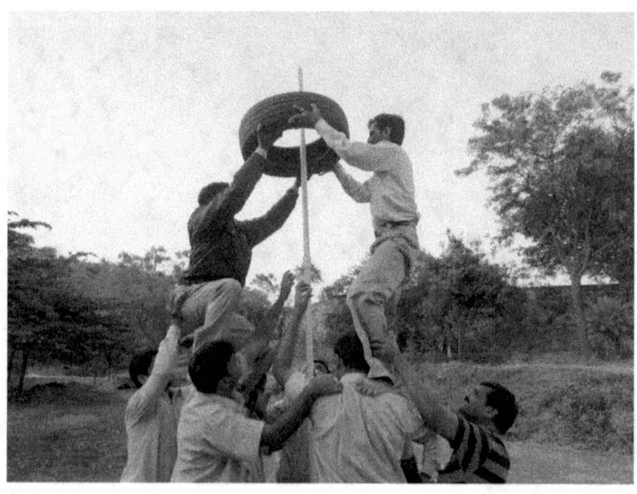

Rapelling down the mountain:
Team work, Confidence building, Achievement, Motivation, Risk taking and Safety.

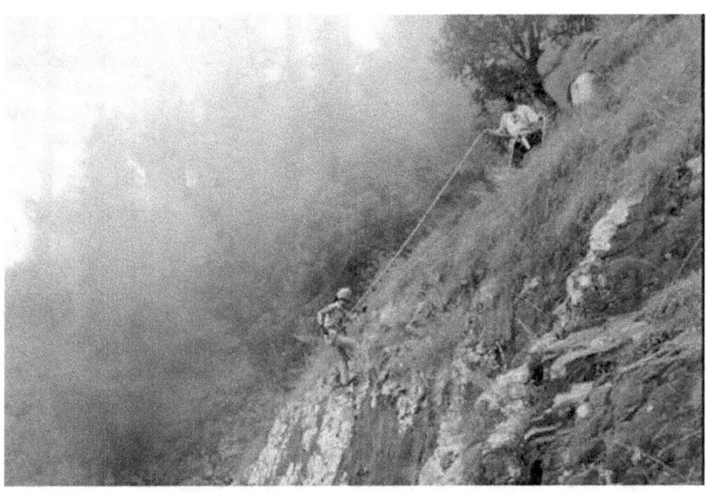

Taking the body across:
Team work, Carefully examining and arranging the team, Encourage and Support .

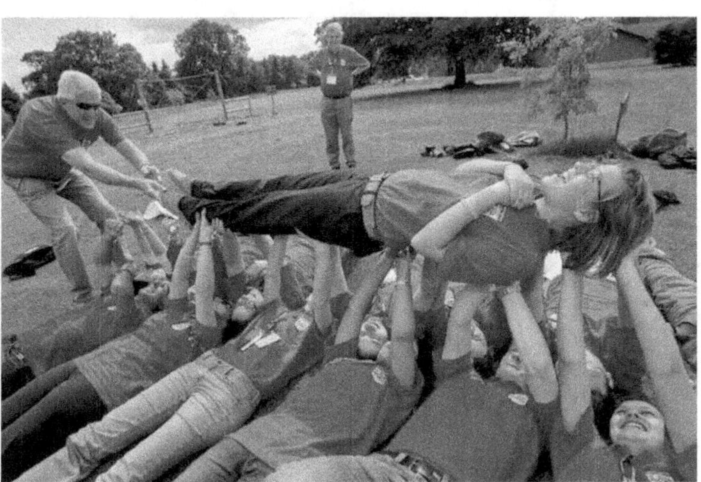

Tackling 12 feet wall:
Strategic planning, Team work, Communication, Support, Encourage and Make judgment.

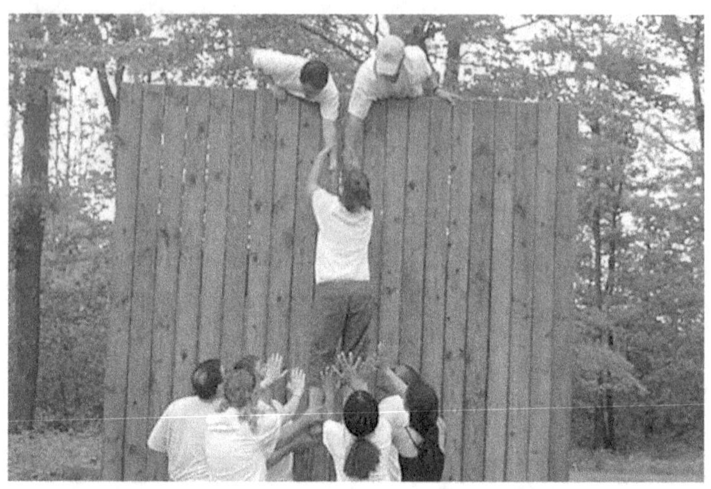

Tug of war:
Motivate, Encourage, Support, Using the resources effectively.

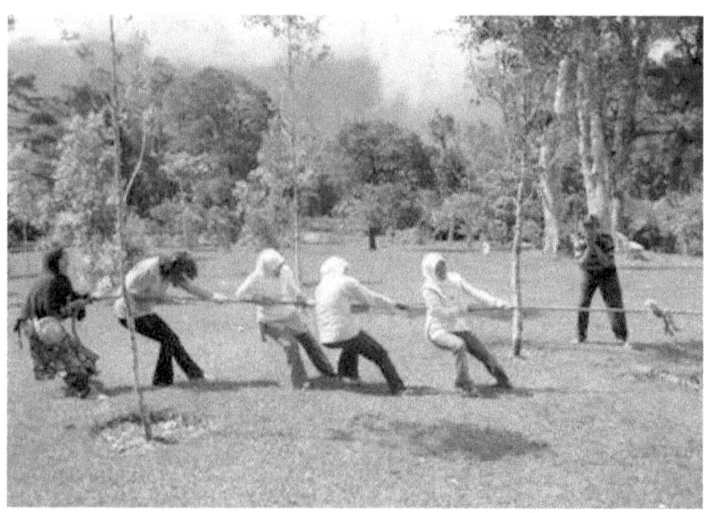

Blindfold walk:

Harder to lead than to follow, Support, Consult, Communicate and Leadership.

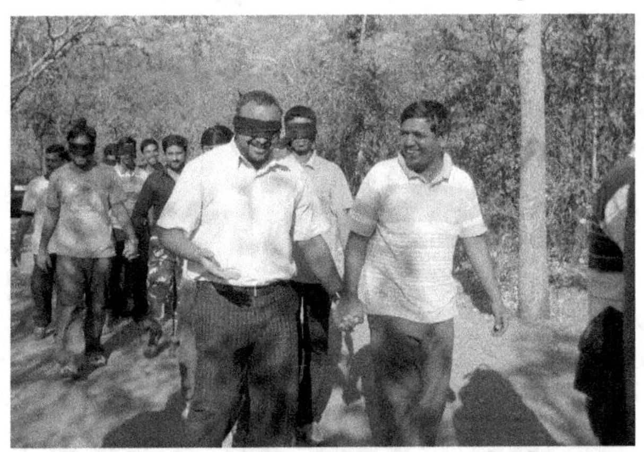

Water chain:

Team work, Support, Consult, plan and Control the leakage.

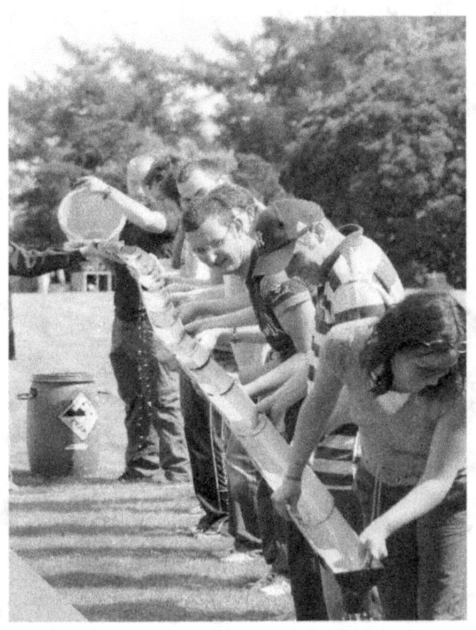

River crossing:

Risk taking, Impotence of safety, Support, Motivate and Encourage.

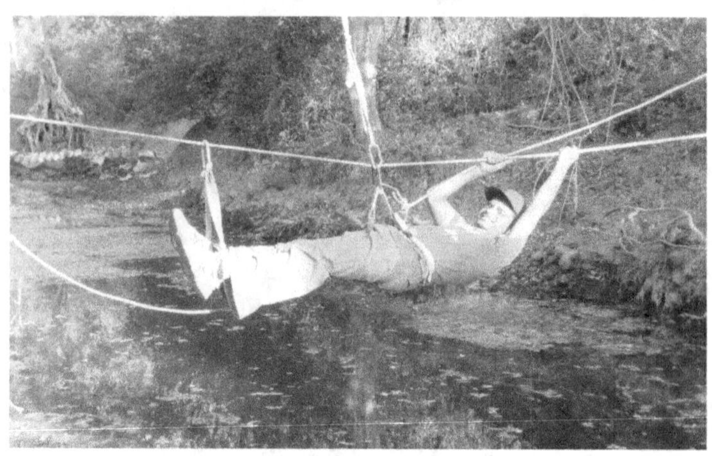

Jump and catch the rope:

Reach-stretch yourself, Risk taking, Confidence building, Make judgment, Monitor and Control.

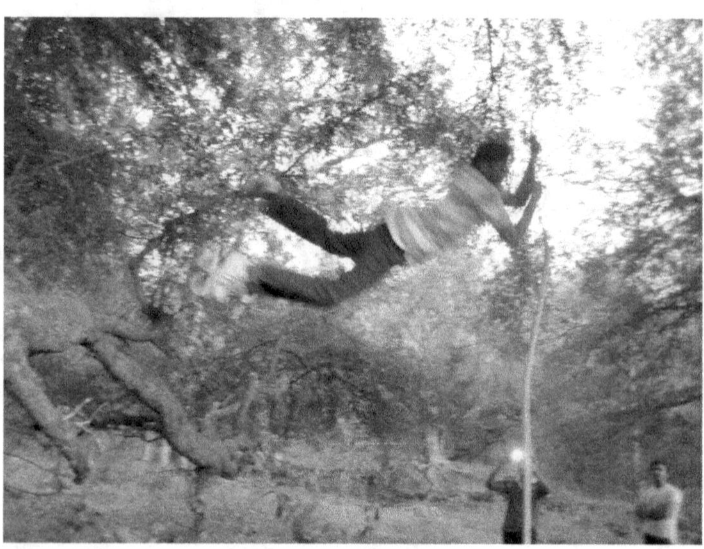

12. Know before you swing into action!

Hundreds of corporations send employees to participate in adventure based programs. But risk conscious business executives find the thrill terrifying. The mystique surrounding these activities spawns vision of million dollar lawsuits and deters many from program participation or sponsorship. Corporate sponsors of adventure programs may minimize risk of injury to participants and reduce risk of lawsuit by identifying relevant legal issues carefully selecting program providers and giving attention to the safety aspects of program activities. Well run adventure activities are often safer than much regular recreational activities.

The sheer thrill of rock climbing, river running, survival trekking, pole climbing and other outdoor activities is responsible for much of the success of adventure enhanced management development programs, Hundreds of corporations send employees to participate in these programs. But risk conscious business executives find the thrill terrifying. The mystique surrounding these activities spawns vision of million dollar lawsuits and deters many from program participation or sponsorship.

Adventure Training Benefits:

Adventure programs enhance personal awareness and provide decision making opportunities in a dynamic stressful environment. For example, one adventure learning provider Outward Bound deliberately places their participants in "stressful" situations that challenge them to overcome obstacles that appear dangerous and perhaps impossible but actually are safe and highly conquerable. Many believe that the personal challenge of adventure activities helps overcome conventional thinking.

Almost all adventure learning activities happen outdoors and use physical activity to teach problem solving, time management, communication, planning, team participation, leadership and interpersonal skills. These activities require intense teamwork and they can improve participants self-esteem and enhance their interpersonal skills... The idea that these experiences build personal confidence and willingness to trust others.

Many organizations offer adventures management development training. Outward Bound which evolved from British wartime survival schools offers it's Corporate Development Program. Boston University's Executive Challenge Program teaches problem solving under stressful conditions. Executive Adventure Inc. models Boston University program. Other providers include the National Outdoor Leadership School, Vermont Voyageur Expeditions and the Mountaineering School at Vail. The American Alpine Institute, River Travel Center Colorado Adventure network and the Pecos River Ranch and Learning Center also offer programs. Some organization such as the Norton Company use outdoor activities as part of their in house training.

Liability Concerns:

Dramatic headlines and publicized incidents cause concern among business executives considering sponsorship of adventure programs. According to a November 23, 1979. Washington Post Article, one lawsuit charged South west Outward Bound with failure to provide adequate supervision, leadership basic skills, training, weather information, safety procedures, equipment or rescue aid. A similar suit charged a Colorado organization with negligence in the death of a program participant Nine of 11 people died on a trip sponsored by an Oregon School in 1986. The two survivors suffered in severe injuries.

These are the exceptions rather than the rule, however In 1986 Outward Bound published a report citing that since 1978, 80,000 people participated in their program with zero fatalities. Injuries ran at 0.70 per 1000 student program days. More than 500 schools universities and organizations safely sponsor adventure activities.

Safety First:

Virtually any situation that results in the death or serious injury of a program participant will lead to litigation. Outdoor activities usually are Subject to state and federal laws including those of the Forest Service, the national Park Service, the Environmental Protection Agency and the Bureau of Land Management. A company is deemed liable because the employees are participating in the wilderness activities as a part of their employment, and the agency or school providing the activities will be considered an independent contractor. Thus successful programs focus on anticipating and preventing participant injury.

An adventure training school or agency should maintain and be eager to provide an accurate record of past incidents that have resulted in fatalities or injuries to program participants. For example Outward Bound USA has an established accident reporting system and prepares and annual safety report to assist its managers in reviewing the safety of the year's program and in charting progress in reducing accidents injuries and illnesses. In addition Outward Bound has instituted a review process whereby its safety program is independently audited every two years.

Since program safety might be an issue in future litigation a professional program provider should be able to substantiate its safety record using data obtained from accident report forms. Accident report forms should be kept on file and be available upon request.

Safety management constitutes the plans the daily decisions and the actions taken by providers to ensure minimum risk to trainees, Program design, safety procedures, organizational structure, emergency planning and qualifications of staff are essential features to examine when evaluating a providers demeanor towards safety issues. A good safety record dose not just happen. It is the result of deliberate planning for safety.

Sense and Sensibility:

Common sense requires program directors to anticipate and minimize unnecessary risks and the law requires no less. This rule applies to all types of outdoor activities from company picnics to rock climbing expeditions. The law applies "the reasonable and prudent person standard" to all recreation activities not just high adventure programs. This standard is applied to determine if the defendant acted as a reasonable person should be expected to act under similar circumstances. Negligence is ruled if the defendant's actions fall below that standard. In the April 1978 Journal of Physical Educations and Recreation Janna Rankin suggests that adventure activity risks may be even lower than risks for traditional recreation because adventure activities require extra care which reduces injury levels. Moreover, the visible danger motivates participants to follow directions more closely.

Most lawsuits assert two grounds for liability:

- Negligence in program selection, planning or operation,
- Strict liability for dangerous activities.

Negligence:

Negligence is a tort – a civil wrong – based on moral fault. Negligence is a careless violation of the rights or privileges of another. While society condemns carelessness less than intended injury to another, careless people must pay for the injuries they cause. Injuries include those to property as well as those to people Negligence requires proof of four elements.

- Legal duty
- Breach of duty
- Breach of duty caused the injury.
- Injury

Duty:

Duty is the most important element in a tort action Legislative enactments or government regulations may establish duties. For example the Occupational safety and Health Administration (OSHA) regulations specify safety standards in the workplace in the absence of specific guidelines, however, conduct must conform to that of a reasonable and prudent person. Courts use common sense to determine reasonable behavior under the circumstances of the case. The specific categories of duty follow.

Professional care:

Recreation program leaders should exercise the care expected of any reasonable and prudent person. Adventure program leaders, however often must exercise extraordinary care because they supervise activities with little room for error. Courts require reasonable and prudent professional supervision. Courts measure leader conduct against other adventure program leaders rather than against regular recreation leaders. Expert witness help the court determine if a leader's behavior is professional. This means providing adequate instruction proper supervision, safe and adequate equipment and a safe activity site.

Any area or site in which a program activity is conducted should be potentially safe and appropriate for the nature of the activity. It should provide the resources to meet the needs of the activity and not pose hazards that create unnecessary risks for participants.

Formal orientation of trainees is a critical part of the safety of an adventure management development program. Prior to the start of activities participants should be trainees in the skills needed for the wilderness experience. The training should include "practice runs" so the staff can supervise the performance of the trainees" readiness and ensure adequate instruction. Participants should be told of potential hazards and be taught proper techniques for dealing with them.

Nearly every aspect of an adventure training program depends on some type of specialized equipment. Instruction should assure that participants know what the equipment is, what it is used for and how to properly use. Maintain, and inspect it.

The program provider also should have established rules and regulations to govern the participants conduct and to delineate acceptable and unacceptable behavior. Each participant should get a copy of these rules.

Duty to prevent or mitigate injury. Usually the law only required people to refrain from conduct that may injure another. Occasionally however the law requires action to prevent or mitigate harm to another. Any legally recognized relationship with the potential victim may compel a reasonable rescue attempt. For example parents must make reasonable efforts to rescue a child from perilous circumstances. Similarly a school district owes adequate supervision to student participants in a wrestling match. Likewise adventure program leaders must make reasonable rescue attempts regardless of the reason for the peril.

Accidents sometimes occur regardless of the care or precautions taken by the agency or school. A review of the emergency procedures of a safe adventure training program should reveal that the program is equipped and well prepared to cope with emergencies in a prompt and professional manner. Arrangement for emergencies should include coordination with groups capable of providing emergency medical services, rescue teams and hospitals.

Leadership should anticipate participant errors. They must plan and trained for rescue operation they need to carefully monitor participants and their progress to the activity. Finally, they must make reasonable efforts to get people out of danger, regardless of the source of danger.

Because reporting forms focus on critical safety aspects of adventure training, it is wise to review all such forms used by the program provider. First aid forms authorized medical treatment but they also established the participants. Perception of his or her present medical condition. But a first aid forms does not substitute for the record of a medical examination which should be required of all participants – especially when activities will be strenuous. The first aid forms should contained a simple authorization clause for medical treatment if needed and should request information about any physical conditions that may affect performance, any prescription drugs being used, the name of one's insurance company, the identification number of the policy, and the name of the contact person in case of an emergency.

Activity selection and design

Answers to the following questions established the reasonableness of an activities risk

- What does the activity risk? Note that people are more valuable than property.
- Why did the person assume risk? E.g. was participation knowing and voluntary or because instructor applied pressure?
- How significant is the risk? Is the potential for injury a bruised ego or broken bones?
- What purpose does the risk serve? How does exposure to the risk help people?
- How necessary is the risk? Can other activity produce the same result without the risk?

Activity currency:

Adventure activities, because of inherent danger, require careful and attentive supervision. The ability to foresee danger may be the key to accident prevention. Trained professionals have greater ability to plan for an foresee danger. Activity design must be current and leaders must use the best current. Practices for the activity. Dangerous activities of course, require more care and currency. Finally, providers of adventure training should be able to provide evidence that the supervisor and instructional staff are highly qualified well trained and technically skilled.

Safety procedures:

Participants put complete trust in activity leaders, who should make every efforts to participant safely. Complete trust in the activity instructor should anticipate and sense dangerous situations and prepared to deal with potential problems. They should also anticipate participants' reaction to stressful situations. As the adage warns, an ounce of prevention is worth a pound of cure in adventure activities, an ounce of safety may save a life or thousands of dollars in legal damages.

Causation:

Causation means that the injury results from some action or lack of action by a careless person. It is an unbroken chain of events leading from the careless act to the injury. If injuries result from several contributing causes, the courts divide the financial responsibility among the careless parties based on degree of fault.

Sometimes another event reinforces or supersedes the consequences of original carelessness. This "intervening cause" alters the sequence of events Liability shifts to the actor setting the intervening chain of causality in motion. For example a rock climber slips because of negligent supervision by the instructor. Then safety equipment fails because of a product defect. The safety equipment manufacturer would pay most injury costs.

If a reasonable person would have foreseen undesirable consequences from an action the provider must pay It does not matter what specific harms foreseen. If potential for harm is foreseeable,liability follows the action. Given the "moral fault" logic of negligence, this rule excludes liability for extraordinary and unpreventable events. For example a ship painter who accidently drops a cigarette into a can of paint must pay for damage to the painting equipment. He would not pay however for damage to the ship dock and town that burns as well.

Activity leader should foresee consequences related to the learning site for example injuries from a fall or falling rocks at a site with loose rock. The same guideline applies to participants abilities. Professionals should foresee injuries to participants maneuvering without preparation.

Injuries

Courts require proof of injury as part of a negligence claim. An injury is any invasion of some legally protected right or interest. Punitive damages occur when a total disregard for the interest of others is demonstrated Punitive damages punish the defendant either to prevent him from doing the act again or to set an example for others. Injuries in adventure programs can include frostbite, hypothermia, broken bones and injuries from falls or falling rock. Compensation should place the victim in the same economic position as if no injury had occurred. Damages are awarded for medical expenses and lost wages as well as for pain and suffering. The damages must be reasonably certain in amount. Contrary to popular belief the courts do not speculate on the damage suffered by a person. The injured person must introduce credible evidence supporting the damage claim. Medical experts predict the probability for recovery and course of treatment. Economics estimate loss of earning power due to injuries.

Often a participant's injuries result from his own carelessness or inattention. Traditionally this contributory negligence prevents recovery of damages for the negligence to any other person. The "last clear chance" doctrine softens this rule. It assigns financial responsibility to the party with the last clear chance of preventing the injuries.

Today most states have replaced the contributory negligence and last clear chance doctrines with comparative negligence. Under comparative negligence specifications the court distributes responsibility for an accident among the people involved in the accident. Those least culpable pay damages based on the difference between their percentage of fault and the percentage of the other parties.

Assumption of Risk:

The courts recognize that certain activities such as basketball games, have inherent risk that participants assume. They do not however, assume risk beyond those logically related to the activity. A basketball player would e.g. recovered damages for intentional bite by another player.

The assumption of risk defense requires giving participants full information on the nature and potential risks of the activity. The participants must then freely assent to participation in the activity. Written assent is not necessary although a written participation agreement outlining the activities and risks considerably strengthens the credibility of this defense. It is also crucial to avoid any taint of pressure on people to participate. This can be difficult where corporate cultures stress teamwork and conformity to corporate standards.

Leaders should never force or pressurize any person to participate in an activity especially one they cannot physically do. Where participants are forced or pressured to perform an activity and some injury results, both the provider and the employer will be legally vulnerable. Thus the program should have an established policy of voluntary participation for trainees.

The courts have indicated that participants not only must be knowledgeable about a danger but that they also must have an appreciation for the danger. This requires instruction regarding all associated risks where they are likely to be present and the potential consequences associated with those risks. Each participants should also be instructed regarding emergency procedures and first aid.

Strict liability:

A strict liability applies to abnormally hazardous conditions or activities. Social policy rather than moral fault forms the basis for assigning liability. The courts reason that those who sponsor hazardous enterprises are better able to bear the risk than the injured. Strict liability actions have fewer elements of proof than negligence actions. Strict liability applies to dangerously defective products, explosives, pesticides, and food and drug products. While strict liability does not generally apply to services. Arthur frank in the April 1978 journal of Physical Education and Recreation cautions that the reference to adventure programs as high risk may cause courts to impose strict liability.

Program provider agreements:

Employers should select providers for adventure programs with the best safety record and qualified staff. Get specific details about the provider such as its injury record, type of program, emergency procedures and orientation activities for participants. Before finally selecting a provider, get enough information to be able to respond to employee's questions regarding program safety.

As companies negotiate agreements for adventure training, liability issues arise. The main issue is discerning how much liability falls on the program sponsor and how much falls on the program providers.

When contracting with a provider of adventure management training programs a firm should obtain a "hold harmless" agreement from the provider. This kind of agreement seeks to wave the company liability for injury illness fatality and public liability. A company also should request supporting documentation that the provider carries adequate liability and medical insurance.

Generally a written agreement details the relationship between program sponsor and program provider including insurance and liability provisions. Despite agreement assigning liability to program providers, sponsors should carefully investigate program safety precautions, scrutinize site selections and make certain that providers have adequate insurance coverage. Sponsors should also examine the safety record and financial viability of program providers. Courts look for deep pockets when grievous injuries occur and inadequate insurance coverage exists. For example a large successful vendor will have deeper pockets when grievous injuries occur and inadequate insurance coverage exists. For example a large successful vendor will have deeper pockets than a nonprofit organization.

Courts use a "control of work" test to determine the nature of the relationship between sponsors and providers. If the sponsor controls the work then the provider is an employee and the sponsor bears liability for the acts of the employee within the scope of employment. If the provider controls the work, the provider becomes an independent contractor and bears the liability. This rule makes sense when applies injuries to customers or by standers resulting from providers negligence. The courts have more difficulty applying the rule when contractors provide services for sponsors' employees. For example an employee in an automobile accident while returning from a company sponsored golf outing. The court determined that the death occurred in the course of employment since the company sponsored arranged and financed the golf outing. Sponsors should examine liability coverage to determine if coverage extends to outings and programs sponsored for employees.

Waiver forms also are referred to as release forms statements of understanding or covenants not to sue. The legal value of these forms varies by jurisdiction and depends to some extent upon the wording. It would be prudent for an organization to have an attorney review and evaluate the waiver form. When participants are informed of the dangers and hazards present in activities, waiver forms may serve as bars against certain types of actions in jurisdictions in which waiver forms are viewed as covenants not to sue rather than as release agreements. If the form is worded correctly, it informs a participant of inherent risk. The waiver form should be signed in the presence of a notary public. Each participant should be allowed sufficient time to read and review the contents before signing otherwise courts may decide that the participants was not fully aware of all the risks involved.

Insurance Benefits:

Many companies offer life disability accident and medical insurance plans. These programs generally cover injuries to employees whether the injury is job related or not although some dangerous activity exclusions might exists. The main issue concerning insurance contracts centers around coordination of benefits clauses. Insurance agreements generally provide that if other insurance coverage exists injured people may not recover more than actual medical expenses. Furthermore the policies prorate benefit payments among insurance companies. In any event the provision of employer paid insurance will frequently reduce the potential for litigation and the amount of eventual judgment in the event of a trail.

Workers Compensation

Worker's compensation systems provide compensation to employees injured on the job regardless if fault. Moreover, these statutes provide some protection to employers against excessive liability. Work-related activities may include attendance at and travel to or from employer – sponsored activities. The courts will use the following issues to determine if an activity is work related.

- Did the employer pressure the employee to attend the function?

- Does sponsorship of the activity benefit the employer?

- To what extent did the employer sponsor, control, of participate in the activity?

- If the activity constitutes a benefit of consideration paid to the employee, such as activities awarded as sales prizes, worker's compensation does not apply.

Recent court decisions disclose a trend of extending benefits to employees injured while attending or traveling to or from employer sponsored training program.

Development for today's organization

Human resources drive today's information society. Organizations successful in developing their human resources achieve market advantages by creating environments that stimulate. Personal and professional employee growth. These environments attract bright, creative, intelligent employees. In *Reinventing the Corporation* John Naisbett suggests that thinking,learning and creating are the most important skills in our information based society. Adventure management development programs offer business a new alternative for teaching these skills. These programs use activities to promote team building communications, creativity and reasonable risk taking.

Business sponsorship of adventure programs has increased in recent years These programs have more visible danger than traditional training Suggestions for improving the safety of such programs include the following.

- Obtain adequate health histories and where appropriate physical examinations of participants.

- Provide current step by step instruction. Make sure participants feel comfortable using equipment.

- Do not pressure reluctant participants to continue the activity.

- Foresee and avoid hazardous site conditions.

- Explain risks and hazards before starting the activity.

- Understand how people react to stress and assist those with inappropriate reactions in safety completing the activity.

- Sponsors should be informed about the legal risks to these programs and should choose or design their programs with safety in mind. This safety focus reduces the legal risk of such activities.

13. Evaluation: Physical-Intellectual-Emotional.

Evaluation should become an essential part of the training process. This however does not mean that a "one size fits all" approach is appropriate. Organization needs to accept that this is an important stage in the overall learning and development process.

The most elementary reason for providing training is to explore opportunities for the development and also to ensure that an employee is able to carry out their current role which would be in sync to the organization's goals and objectives. Organization believes that adding value to the employee will benefit in having highly skilled and acknowledgeable employees.

Organizations which are keen to increase their productivity, efficiency and profitability will look to move beyond obligatory and traditional training methods and look at more diverse and innovative learning and development practices which will enable the employees to capitalize on their potential and prove to be a valuable resource for the organization. Outdoor learning activities can be a source where employees gain new knowledge and skills, which provides a strong argument for organizations to invest in their employees so that they can benefit and differentiate themselves from their competitors.

Opportunities need to be appropriate in terms of contents and the way it is delivered so that they will add value to the employees and the overall organization. Most important is learning outdoor activities need to be delivered in such a way that practical benefits to the workplace can be observed, along with enabling employees to be able to transfer their new knowledge and skills to the benefit of all of the key stakeholders.

Training programmes are effective only to the extend that the skills and behaviors learned and practiced are actually transferred to the workplace.

It is extremely important that the employees need to be actively aware of an organization's strategies and objectives and the fact that learning opportunities can help to strengthen this.

What do you mean by evaluation of learning and development?

Training evaluation can be defined as a systematic process of collecting and analyzing information for and about a training programme which can be used for planning and influencing decision making as well as assessing the relevance, effectiveness and the impact of various training components.

James and Roffe provide a simplified explanation of evaluation "Comparing the actual and real with the predicted or promised" which emphasizes the need to reflect on what was achieved in comparison to what was expected for. This definition also highlights that potential for different individuals are likely to have diverse expectations and their review of the events may also differ depending on a wide range of variables. Dawson provides another explanation which suggests that the process should be impartial and devoid of subjective opinion: The evaluation of training is the systematic and impartial collection of data for managers and all other interested parties. This information equips them to draw conclusions about the effectiveness of particular training measures as a way of achieving organizational objectives, implementing policy and promoting organizational learning.

The importance of evaluating learning and development activities:

Mann states "with the huge investment in developing training strategies, the question is no longer 'should we train' but rather "is the training worthwhile and effective?"

For the organization:

There are number of reasons why organizations should evaluate their learning and development activities

- To make help decisions about what interventions should be or should not be duplicated in the future.
- To establish the value that interventions bring to the organizations.
- As a part of business efficiency considerations.
- To reinforce the importance of an evaluation process when testing new programmes for employees.
- To assist in determining who should attend training programmes.
- To allow the organization to identify better ways to achieve things rather than through the provision of formal learning interventions.

For the individuals:

Evaluation gives employees with opportunity to give feedback to their trainers. Individuals can also benefit from the evaluation process if feedback is acted upon for the benefit of the programme.

For trainers/facilitators:

Evaluation data may be used as a performance indicator which justifies the presence of training department and/ or investment in trainers. Independent trainers may also depend on their feedback to gain future business and /or to engage with potential new clienteles as an indicator of the quality of their provision and delivery.

The purpose of evaluation

1. Assess if proposed learning objectives have been met.

2. Continuous enhancement of learning interventions.

3. Assess whether resources are used judiciously.

4. Asses the value for money of the learning interventions.

Linking learning, development and evaluation to business strategy:

Learning can provide a crucial link between an organization's human resource strategy and overall business strategy by ensuring that the organization's employees have the relevant skills and knowledge need to be able to execute the HR strategy. As the strategies are updated it will be necessary to review the learning and development process and therefore an ongoing dialogue is needed between those responsible for learning and senior management.

Models of evaluation:

The Kirkpatrick Model.: In 1960s Donald Kirkpatrick wrote a series of articles on evaluation where he identified four stages or levels of evaluation. Despite its age, Kirkpatrick model continues to be used in contemporary research. Kirkpatrick divided the evaluation process into four segments or stages.

Stage One – Reaction How do the participants feel about the programme they attended?

Stage Two – Learning To what extent have the trainees learned the information and skills?

Stage Three – Behavior To what extent have their job behavior changed as a result of attending the training programme?

Stage Four – Results To what extent have results been affected by the training program?

Cheng and Hampson [2008] argue that levels three and four are not often used because organizations find it much simpler just to focus on the first two levels. Alliger and Janak [1989] argue that some interventions will not aim to meet all four levels and this does not necessarily mean that it should not be used; assuming it meets the required needs. This highlights the clear need for organizations to consider what form of evaluation is needed to accept that for some programmers, evaluation at stages one and two may provide sufficient information.

Alternative model: The CIRO [**C**ontext, **I**nput, **R**eaction, **O**utcome] model focuses on three questions and the main difference from Kirkpatrick model is that it focuses on measurements taken before and after the training has been carried out. Perhaps the key strength of this model is that it takes in to account the resources of the organization [with in the input measure] and their objectives [within the context measure] thereby responding to some of the criticisms of Kirkpatrick. Tennate et al critique this model by highlighting that it does not take behavior in to account they also believe that it is suitable for managerial focused training programme rather than those that are less specialized and perhaps aimed at people working at low levels in the organizations.

The CIRO approach to evaluate training impact is four level approach which was originally developed by Warr, Bird and Racham.

Context evaluation	What needs to be addressed?
Input evaluation	What is likely to bring about the changes?
Reaction evaluation	How did the learners react to the training?
Outcome evaluation	What are immediate, intermediate and ultimate Outcomes?

Context evaluation:

It involves collecting information about performance deficiency, assessing that information to establish training needs and on the basis of those findings, setting of objectives. Context of the learning event concerns with procuring and using information about the current functional situation in order to determine training needs and objectives. This evaluation determines if training is needed. During this process three types of objectives may be evaluated.

Input evaluation:

It concerns with how well the learning intervention was planned, organized, designed and delivered. It involves determining cost efficiency and cost effectiveness and feasibility. It involves analyzing the available resources and determining how they can be developed in order to achieve desired objectives.

Reaction evaluation:

It concerns with obtaining and using information about participants' reactions to improve the intervention. The distinguishing feature of this type of evaluation is that it relies on subjective inputs of participants. This can be helpful when collected and used in systematic and objective manner.

Outcome evaluation:

This involves assessing what actually happened as a result of learning event. This can be seen as changes in participants' knowledge., skills and attitudes, comparing it the beginning and at the completion of the training. At workplace level this can be measured by appraisal, observation, discussion with the manager of learner/peers/customers/clients. The team/departmental level: It involves identifying changes that take place in team, department or unit as a result of learning event. Changes at departmental level may include change in the departmental output, costs, clash rates, absentism, staff turnover etc. The changes which may occur after the introduction of training programme may include change in culture of organization, more flexibility, and reduced level of conflict, enhanced ability to attract and retain valued workers.

Outward Bound Learning for mergers of 3 companies: a case study -

Media companies had lately gone through a series of mergers and joint ventures to form **"Media works."** It was an amalgamation of 3 companies put together of learning initiatives at merger of three television media companies was evaluated by putting them under experiential learning outdoor exercises.

There were newly appointed leaders and business heads. The HR heads and the CEO realized that a cohesive team would have to be built to take the business ahead. The three different organizations had different cultures, policies, processes and working styles, varied demographics, geographical locations etc. The task at hand was to show a substantial growth due to merger of three companies. A meeting was held between the business heads and HR heads to evaluate the situation and suggest appropriate measures to tackle the situation.

The discussion recognized the current problem areas, the suggestive steps to be taken, and desired results expected. After a brief study and research done, it was decided that Outward Bound learning intervention would be suitable for addressing the situation. Series of meetings were held with business heads. Each region would go on an offsite with the respective cross functional teams. This would help the respective teams. Understand each other's function; understand the behaviors and personality of their colleagues, since the team members were based out of different geographical locations. It would give a team an opportunity to bond with each other and understand each other better. As the leaders were newly appointed, the leader would have his entire team together to understand each one's strength, areas to be developed, operational issues etc. On the other hand the team members would also be able to gauge the expectations of the leader, and the working styles.

The offsite location was chosen keeping in mind factors like, minimum travel time, and logistic issues. The location would be on the outskirts of the city, as it would help the team be in a natural environment, without external disturbances. A four day programme was conducted in the Reserve forest with activities revolving around experiential learning. The programme was designed and facilitated to address the issues or concerns. This was followed by reflections and observation which were internalized as leanings which would be implemented in the future activities as well as at the workplace.

Context evaluation:

What needs to be addressed?

At Media works, the CEO along with the HR head identified the broad problem of team cohesiveness. As the new company was a merger and joint venture for three companies, many organizational and cultural problems were creeping up. There was lot of discontent within the team, and they were working like a mini organizations competing against each other. To have more clarity and focus on the problem, a separate meeting was held with the business heads and the HR heads present. This helped in breaking down the problem and identifying the exact issues. Some of the issues which needed to be addressed on priority were

- The team being cohesive.
- The interaction and understanding between cross functional teams to be addressed.
- As the leaders were newly appointed, the department heads were to have a complete look at the new team members. Understanding the new team demographics,

the strengths and areas of developmental each team member, understanding the operational issues, mentoring them on the business objectives etc. were a few of the things which needed immediate attention from the leaders point of view.

- The team members also wanted to know their leader, understand his style of working, expectations of the leaders etc.

- As the team was based out of different geographical locations, they needed to emphasize, coordinate and work as team.

Limitations:

* A survey could have been done internally within the region to understand the expectations and the requirements of the team members too.

* An external agency could have been appointed to do a climate check of the organization and give a different view to the whole problem.

Input evaluation

What is likely to bring about the changes?

The OBET or the experiential learning intervention was chosen based on the studies and research done on the different types of HR interventions suitable to address the issues. The location chosen was away from the city in the reserve forest to let the participants get a complete exposure to the natural environment, without any external interruptions. The outdoor experience and setting was to give the team members maximum exposure to the natural environment, spend time together, and perform activities entrusted etc. Experiential learning was suited for this as the activities and the programme was designed keeping in mind the issues to be addressed. The health, safety and physical conditions of the participants were also considered while designing the training programme. An external facilitator was shortlisted based on their experience, industry knowledge, safety and facilities available to host the training programme.

Experiential learning was seen a four stage cycle

1. Concrete personal experience, followed by
2. Observation of the reflection upon one's experiences, which leads to
3. Formation of generalizations and earnings, leading to
4. Hypothesis to be tested by future actions, which in turn leads to new experiences.

Reaction evaluation

How did the learners react to the training?

The participants and the team members were very happy and welcomed the new methods of intervention without any prejudices. The natural environment with natural surroundings helped in breaking the ice among team members. As the agenda was different from the usual business matters, the team members discuss and worked together as a team to accomplish the tasks given. Initially the team began with lot of apprehensions and reservations but as the activities and the tasks progressed the team began to loosen up and understand the underlying reason and objective of the entire training programme.

The leaders also played their role effectively, guiding, mentoring the team wherever required. Towards the end of the training, a formal feedback was taken from participants. Majority of the participants were happy and satisfied with the training programme, the design of the programme, the activities, the facilities provided etc. The team members also acknowledged that the experiential style of learning was beneficial and was appropriate for maximum learning.

Outcome evaluation

What are the immediate, intermediate and ultimate outcomes?

The outcome of training was visible right from the time the training began. There was more bonding and cohesiveness among the team. With in three months period, the internal grievances had dropped considerably. The relationship between the cross functional teams improved, which directly impacted the turnaround time, the efficiency and the productivity. At an individual level, a sense of belongingness towards the organization was seen. Individuals were more relaxed and focused on the job profile entrusted. At the workplace, there were fewer scraps amongst team members; they were more co-operative, cohesive. Overall at the organizational level there was a complete transformation in the organization culture. All the departments worked as a single unit, towards the organizational goals and objectives. This was proven by the performance and turnover of the organization which grew significantly.

14. Opening themselves to others!

Ingham and Luft's Johari Window model is for self-awareness, personal development, group development and understanding relationships. Today the Johari Window model is especially relevant due to modern emphasis on, and influence of, 'soft' skills, behavior, empathy, cooperation, inter-group development and interpersonal development. The Johari Window concept is particularly helpful to understanding employee/employer relationships within the Psychological Contract.

The Johari Window model is a simple and useful tool for illustrating and improving self-awareness, and mutual understanding between individuals within a group. The Johari Window model can also be used to assess and improve a group's relationship with other groups. The Johari Window model was devised by American psychologists Joseph Luft and Harry Ingham in 1955, while researching group dynamics at the University of California Los Angeles. The model was first published in the Proceedings of the Western Training Laboratory in Group Development by UCLA Extension Office in 1955, and was later expanded by Joseph Luft. Today the Johari Window model is especially relevant due to modern emphasis on, and influence of, 'soft' skills, behavior, empathy, cooperation, inter-group development and interpersonal development.

The Johari Window concept is particularly helpful to understanding employee/employer relationships within the Psychological Contract.

Over the years, alternative Johari Window terminology has been developed and adapted by other people – particularly leading to different descriptions of the four regions, hence the use of different terms in this explanation. Don't let it all confuse you – the Johari Window model is really very simple indeed.

Luft and Ingham called their Johari Window model 'Johari' after combining their first names, Joe and Harry. In early publications the word appears as 'JoHari'. The Johari Window soon became a widely used model for understanding and training self-awareness, personal development, improving communications, interpersonal relationships, group dynamics, team development and inter-group relationships.

The Johari Window model is also referred to as a 'disclosure/feedback model of self-awareness', and by some people an 'information processing tool'. The Johari Window actually represents information – feelings, experience, views, attitudes, skills, intentions, motivation, etc – within or about a person – in relation to their group, from four perspectives, which are described below. The Johari Window model can also be used to represent the same information for a group in relation to other groups. Johari Window terminology refers to 'self' and 'others': 'self' means oneself, i.e., the person subject to the Johari Window analysis. 'Others' mean other people in the person's group or team.

When the Johari Window model is used to assess and develop groups in relation to other groups, the 'self' would be the group, and 'others' would be other groups. However, for ease of explanation and understanding of the Johari Window and examples in this article, think of the model applying to an individual within a group, rather than a group relating to other groups.

The four Johari Window perspectives are called 'regions' or 'areas' or 'quadrants'. Each of these regions contains and represents the information – feelings, motivation, etc – known about the person, in terms of whether the information is known or unknown by the person, and whether the information is known or unknown by others in the group.

The Johari Window's four regions, (areas, quadrants, or perspectives) are as follows, showing the quadrant numbers and commonly used names:

Johari window four regions

1.   What is known by the person about him/herself and is also known by others – **open area, open self, free area, free self, or 'the arena'**

2.   What is unknown by the person about him/herself but which others know – **blind area, blind self, or 'blind spot'**

3.   What the person knows about him/herself that others do not know – **hidden area, hidden self, avoided area, avoided self or 'facade'**

4.   What is unknown by the person about him/herself and is also unknown by others – **unknown area or unknown self**

Johari window four regions – model diagram

Like some other behavioral models (eg, Tuckman, Hersey/Blanchard), the Johari Window is based on a four-square grid – the Johari Window is like a window with four 'panes'. Here's how the Johari Window is normally shown, with its four regions.

1 open/free area	2 blind area
3 hidden area	4 unknown area

This is the standard representation of the Johari Window model, showing each quadrant the same size.

The Johari Window 'panes' can be changed in size to reflect the relevant proportions of each type of 'knowledge' of/ about a particular person in a given group or team situation.

In new groups or teams the open free space for any team member is small (see the Johari Window new team member example below) because shared awareness is relatively small.

As the team member becomes better established and known, so the size of the team member's open free area quadrant increases. See the Johari Window established team member example below.

Johari quadrant 1 – 'open self/area' or 'free area' or 'public area', or 'arena'

Johari region 1 is also known as the 'area of free activity'. This is the information about the person – behavior, attitude, feelings, emotion, knowledge, experience, skills, views, etc – **known** by the person ('the self') and **known** by the group ('others').

The aim in any group should always be to develop the 'open area' for every person, because when we work in this area with others we are at our most effective and productive and the group is at its most productive too. The open free area, or 'the arena', can be seen as the space where good communications and cooperation occur, free from distractions, mistrust, confusion, conflict and misunderstanding.

Established team members logically tend to have larger open areas than new team members. New team members start with relatively small open areas because relatively little knowledge about the new team member is shared. The size of the open area can be expanded horizontally into the blind space, by seeking and actively listening to feedback from other group members. Thisprocess is known as 'feedback solicitation'. Also, other group members can help a team member expand their open area by offering feedback, sensitively of course. The size of the open area can also be expanded vertically downwards into the hidden or avoided space by the person's disclosure of information, feelings, etc about him/herself to the group and group members. Also, group members can help a person expand their open area into the hidden area by asking the person about him/herself. Managers and team leaders can play an important role in facilitating feedback and disclosure among group members, and indirectly giving feedback to individuals about their own blind areas. Leaders also have a big responsibility to promote a culture and expectation for open, honest, positive, helpful, constructive, sensitive communications, and the sharing of knowledge throughout their organization. Top performing groups, departments, companies and organizations always tend to have a culture of open positive communication, so encouraging the positive development of the 'open area' or 'open self' for everyone is a simple yet fundamental aspect of effective leadership.

Johari quadrant 2 – 'blind self' or 'blind area' or 'blind spot'

Johari region 2 is what is **known** about a person by others in the group, but is **unknown** by the person him/herself. By seeking or soliciting feedback from others, the aim should be to reduce this area and thereby to increase the open area (see the Johari Window diagram below), i.e., to increase self-awareness. This blind area is not an effective or productive space for individuals or groups. This blind area could also be referred to as ignorance about oneself, or issues in which one is deluded. A blind area could also include issues that others are deliberately withholding from a person. We all know how difficult it is to work well when kept in the dark. No-one works well when subject to 'mushroom management'. People who are 'thick-skinned' tend to have a large 'blind area'.

Group members and managers can take some responsibility for helping an individual to reduce their blind area – in turn increasing the open area – by giving sensitive feedback and encouraging disclosure. Managers should promote a climate of non-judgmental feedback, and group response to individual disclosure, which reduces fear and therefore encourages both processes to happen. The extent to which an individual seeks feedback, and the issues on which feedback is sought, must always be at the individual's own discretion. Some people are more resilient than others – care needs to be taken to avoid causing emotional upset. The process of soliciting serious and deep feedback relates to the process of 'self-actualization' described in **Maslow's Hierarchy of Needs development and motivation model.**

Johari quadrant 3 – 'hidden self' or 'hidden area' or 'avoided self/area' or 'facade'

Johari region 3 is what is **known** to ourselves but kept hidden from, and therefore **unknown**, to others. This hidden or avoided self represents information, feelings, etc, anything that a person knows about him/her self, but which is not revealed or is kept hidden from others. The hidden area could also include sensitivities, fears, hidden agendas, manipulative intentions, and secrets – anything that a person knows but does not reveal, for whatever reason. It's natural for very personal and private information and feelings to remain hidden, indeed, certain information, feelings and experiences have no bearing on work, and so can and should remain hidden. However, typically, a lot of hidden information is not very personal, it is work- or performance-related, and so is better positioned in the open area.

Relevant hidden information and feelings, etc, should be moved into the open area through the process of 'disclosure'. The aim should be to disclose and expose relevant information and feelings – hence the Johari Window terminology 'self-disclosure' and 'exposure process', thereby increasing the open area. By telling others how we feel and other information about ourselves we reduce the hidden area, and increase the open area, which enables better understanding, cooperation, trust, team-working effectiveness and productivity. Reducing hidden areas also reduces the potential for confusion, misunderstanding, poor communication, etc, which all distract from and undermine team effectiveness.

Organizational culture and working atmosphere have a major influence on group members' preparedness to disclose their hidden selves. Most people fear judgment or vulnerability and therefore hold back hidden information and feelings, etc, that if moved into the open area, i.e. known by the group as well, would enhance mutual understanding, and thereby improve group awareness, enabling better individual performance and group effectiveness.

The extent to which an individual discloses personal feelings and information, and the issues which are disclosed, and to whom, must always be at the individual's own discretion. Some people are more keen and able than others to disclose. People should disclose at a pace and depth that they find personally comfortable. As with feedback, some people are more resilient than others – care needs to be taken to avoid causing emotional upset. Alsoas with soliciting feedback, the process of serious disclosure relates to the process of 'self-actualization' described in Maslow's Hierarchy of Needs development and motivation model.

Johari quadrant 4 – 'unknown self' or 'area of unknown activity' or 'unknown area'

Johari region 4 contains information, feelings, latent abilities, aptitudes, experiences etc, that are **unknown** to the person him/herself and **unknown** to others in the group.

These unknown issues take a variety of forms: they can be feelings, behaviors, attitudes, capabilities, aptitudes, which can be quite close to the surface, and which can be positive and useful, or they can be deeper aspects of a person's personality, influencing his/her behavior to various degrees. Large unknown areas would typically be expected in younger people, and people who lack experience or self-belief.

Examples of unknown factors are as follows, and the first example is particularly relevant and common, especially in typical organizations and teams:

- An ability that is under-estimated or un-tried through lack of opportunity, encouragement, confidence or training.

- A natural ability or aptitude that a person doesn't realize they possess.

- A fear or aversion that a person does not know they have.

- An unknown illness.

- Repressed or subconscious feelings.

- Conditioned behavior or attitudes from childhood.

The processes by which this information and knowledge can be uncovered are various, and can be prompted through self-discovery or observation by others, or in certain situations through collective or mutual discovery, of the sort of discovery experienced on outward bound courses or other deep or intensive group work. Counseling can also uncover unknown issues, but this would then be known to the person and by one other, rather than by a group.

Whether unknown 'discovered' knowledge moves into the hidden, blind or open area depends on who discovers it and what they do with the knowledge, notably whether it is then given as feedback, or disclosed. As with the processes of soliciting feedback and disclosure, striving to discover information and feelings in the unknown is related to the process of 'self-actualization' described in Maslow's Hierarchy of Needs development and motivation model.

Again as with disclosure and soliciting feedback, the process of self-discovery is a sensitive one. The extent and depth to which an individual is able to seek out discover their unknown feelings must always be at the individual's own discretion. Some people are more keen and able than others to do this.

Uncovering 'hidden talents' – that is unknown aptitudes and skills, not to be confused with developing the Johari 'hidden area' – is another aspect of developing the unknown area, and is not so sensitive as unknown feelings. Providing people with the opportunity to try new things, with no great pressure to succeed, is often a useful way to discover unknown abilities, and thereby reduce the unknown area.

Managers and leaders can help by creating an environment that encourages self-discovery, and to promote the processes of self-discovery, constructive observation and feedback among team members. It is a widely accepted industrial fact that the majority of staff in any organization are at any time working well within their potential. Creating a culture, climate and expectation for self-discovery helps people to fulfill more of their potential and thereby to achieve more, and to contribute more to organizational performance.

A note of caution about Johari region 4: The unknown area could also include repressed or subconscious feelings rooted in formative events and traumatic past experiences, which can stay unknown for a lifetime. In a work or organizational context the Johari Window should not be used to address issues of a clinical nature.

Johari window example – increasing open area through feedback solicitation

<table>
<tr><td>1

open/free area</td><td>2

blind area</td></tr>
<tr><td>3

hidden area</td><td>4

unknown area</td></tr>
</table>

This Johari Window model diagram is an example of increasing the open area, by reduction of the blind area, which would normally be achieved through the process of asking for and then receiving feedback.

Feedback develops the open area by reducing the blind area.

The open area can also be developed through the process of disclosure, which reduces the hidden area.

The unknown area can be reduced in different ways: by others' observation (which increases the blind area); by self-discovery (which increases the hidden area), or by mutual enlightenment – typically via group experiences and discussion – which increases the open area as the unknown area reduces.

A team which understands itself – that is, each person having a strong mutual understanding with the team – is far more effective than a team which does not understand each other- that is, whose members have large hidden, blind, and/or unknown areas.

Team members – and leaders – should always be striving to increase their open free areas, and to reduce their blind, hidden and unknown areas.

Non performing team member:

A person represented by the Johari Window example below will not perform to their best potential, and the team will fail to make full use of the team's potential and the person's potential too. Effort should generally be made by the person to increase his/her open free area, by disclosing information about his/her feelings, experience, views, motivation, etc, which will reduce the size of the hidden area, and increase the open free area.

Seeking feedback about the blind area will reduce the blind area, and will increase the open free area. Discovery through sensitive communications, active listening and experience, will reduce the unknown area, transferring in part to the blind, hidden areas, depending on who knows what, or better still if known by the person and others, to the open free area.

New member of the team

Johari window model – example for new team member or member within a new team

<table>
<tr>
<td>1

open/free area</td>
<td>blind area   2</td>
</tr>
<tr>
<td>hidden area

3</td>
<td>unknown area

4</td>
</tr>
</table>

This Johari Window model diagram is an example of a member of a new team or a person who is new to an existing team.

The open free region is small because others know little about the new person.

Similarly the blind area is small because others know little about the new person.

The hidden or avoided issues and feelings are a relatively large area.

In this particular example the unknown area is the largest, which might be because the person is young, or lacking in self-knowledge or belief.

Established member of the team

Johari window example – established team member example

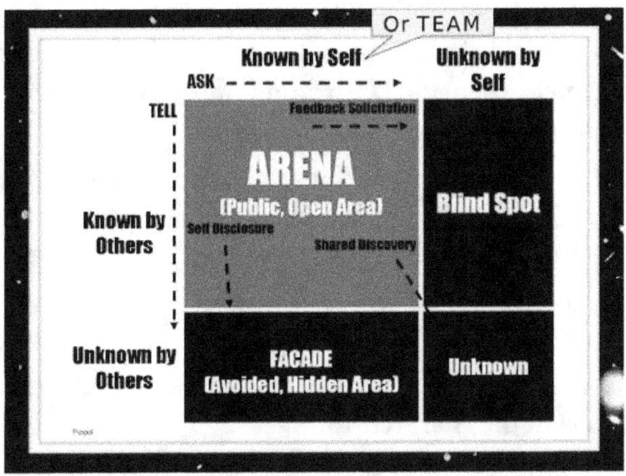

This johari Window model diagram is an example of an established member of a team.

The open free region is large because others know a lot about the person that the person also knows.

Through the processes of disclosure and receiving feedback the open area has expanded and at the same time reduced the sizes of the hidden, blind and unknown areas.

It's helpful to compare the Johari Window model to other four-quadrant behavioral models, notably Bruce Tuckman's **Forming, Storming Norming Performing team development model [Refer Chapter 6]**; also to a lesser but nonetheless interesting extent, The Hersey-Blanchard Situational Leadership team development and management styles model. The common principle is that as the team matures and communications improve, so performance improves too, as less energy is spent on internal issues and clarifying understanding, and more effort is devoted to external aims and productive output.

The Johari Window model also relates to **emotional intelligence theory (EQ)**, and one's awareness and development of emotional intelligence.

As already stated, the Johari Window relates also to Transactional Analysis (notably understanding deeper aspects of the 'unknown' area, region 4).

The Johari Window processes of serious feedback solicitation, disclosure, and striving to uncover one's unknown area relate to Maslow's 'self-actualization' ideas contained in the Hierarchy of Needs.

There are several exercises and activities for Johari Window awareness development among teams featured on the team building games section, for example the ring tones activity.

Exploring more ideas for using Ingham and luft'sJohari window model in training, learning and development

The Johari Window model obviously provides useful background rationale and justification for most things that you might think to do with people relating to developing mutual and self-awareness, all of which links strongly to team effectiveness and harmony.

There are many ways to use the Johari model in learning and development – much as using any other theory such as Maslow's, Tuckman's, TA, NLP, etc. It very much depends on what you want to achieve, rather than approaching the subject from 'what are all the possible uses?' which would be a major investigation.

This being the case, it might help you to ask yourself first what you want to achieve in your training and development activities? And what are your intended outputs and how will you measure that they have been achieved? And then think about how the Johari Window theory and principles can be used to assist this.

Researching academic paperswritten about theories such as Johari is a fertile method of exploring possibilities for concepts and models like Johari. This approach tends to improve your in-depth understanding, instead of simply using specific interpretations or applications 'off-the-shelf', which in themselves might provide good ideas for a one-off session, but don't help you much with understanding how to use the thinking at a deeper level.

Also explore the original work of Ingham and Luft, and reviews of same, relating to the development and applications of the model.

Johari is a very elegant and potent model, and as with other powerful ideas, **simply helping people to understand** is the most effective way to optimize the value to people. Explaining the meaning of the Johari Window theory to people, so they can really properly understand it in their own terms, then empowers people to use the thinking in their own way, and to incorporate the underlying principles into their future thinking and behavior.

Johari window scale

Johari Window [Self Disclosure exercise]

Name: --

Q.1. I am open and candid in my dealings with others as opposed to being closed, conscious and Under wraps in my relationships.

| 1 | 2 | 3 | 4 | 5 | 6 | 7 | 8 | 9 | 10 |

Q.2. I hear, respect and accept the comments and reactions of others As opposed to defensively dismissing them as of little value or turning a deaf Ear on their observations.

| 1 | 2 | 3 | 4 | 5 | 6 | 7 | 8 | 9 | 10 |

Q.3. I specifically test for agreement and commitment to join our team decisions As opposed to assuming that all are committed if no one openly disagrees.

| 1 | 2 | 3 | 4 | 5 | 6 | 7 | 8 | 9 | 10 |

Q.4. I readily admit to confusion or lack of knowledge when I feel that I have little information about the topic under discussion, as opposed, trying to bluff, feigning understanding or Insisting that my opinions are right.

| 1 | 2 | 3 | 4 | 5 | 6 | 7 | 8 | 9 | 10 |

Q.5. I show my concerns that others know where I stand on relevant issues, as opposed to being basically indifferent to others knowledge of me or Just unraveling in my comment.

| 1 | 2 | 3 | 4 | 5 | 6 | 7 | 8 | 9 | 10 |

Q.6. I take the initiative in getting feedback from other members, as opposed to waiting passively for others to offer their comments of their own accord.

| 1 | 2 | 3 | 4 | 5 | 6 | 7 | 8 | 9 | 10 |

Q.7. I leave with others and describe how I feel about what they do and how they do it, as opposedto covering up, taking tolerance or denying any reaction.

> 1   2   3   4   5   6   7   8   9   10

Q. 8. My comments are relevant and pertinent to the real issues at hand in the team, as opposed to being "frothy" or off-target or attempts at camouflage.

> 1   2   3   4   5   6   7   8   9   10

Q. 9. I try to understand how others are feeling and work hard at getting information from them, which will help me do this, as opposed to appearing indifferent, showing superficial concern or being basically insensitive.

> 1   2   3   4   5   6   7   8   9   10

Q.10. I value and encourage reactions equally from others, as opposed To being selective in my quest for feedback to treating some contributions as inferior.

> 1   2   3   4   5   6   7   8   9   10

> 2

Q.11. I am openly affectionate towards others when I feel I like them, as Opposed to being inhibited, restrained or acting embarrassed.

> 1   2   3   4   5   6   7   8   9   10

Q.12. I help others participate and work to support and draw everyone into a group discussion, as opposed to fending only for myself and leaving participation up to Each individual.

> 1   2   3   4   5   6   7   8   9   10

Q.13. I take risks with others and expose highly personal information, both emotional and intellectual when it is pertinent, as opposed to playing it safe, as if I do not trust others.

1   2   3   4   5   6   7   8   9   10

Q.14. I welcome and appreciate other's attempts to help me, no matter how Critical or direct their feed back, as opposed to acting hurt, sulking, indifferent or Rejecting them outright.

1   2   3   4   5   6   7   8   9   10

Q.15. I openly try to influence an individual or a group, as opposed to being Manipulative.

1   2   3   4   5   6   7   8   9   10

3

Q.16. I press for additional information when I am angered by them, asopposed to acting unaffected, restrained or over controlled.

1   2   3   4   5   6   7   8   9   10

Q.17. I am openly hostile towards others when I am angered by them, as Opposed to acting unaffected, restrained, or over controlled.

1   2   3   4   5   6   7   8   9   10

Q.18. I encourage collaboration on problems and solicit others definitions and Solutions on mutual problems, as opposed to insisting on mechanical decision Rules or trying to press my own judgments through.

1   2   3   4   5   6   7   8   9   10

Q.19. I am spontaneous and say what I think no matter how 'far out' it may seem, As opposed to monitoring my contributions so that they are in line with prevailing Through or more acceptable to others.

1   2   3   4   5   6   7   8   9   10

Q.20. I give support to others who are on the spot and struggling to express Themselves intellectually and emotionally, as opposed to letting them flounder or Trying to move on without them.

1   2   3   4   5   6   7   8   9   10

4

SCALE

10	Extremely characteristic	**I do this consistently**
09	Very characteristic	**I do this nearly all the time.**
08	Quite characteristic	**I do this most of the time.**
07	Pretty characteristic	**I do this a good deal of time.**
06	Fairly characteristic	**I do this frequently.**
05	Some what characteristic	**I do this on occasion**
04	Fairly Uncharacteristic	**I seldom do this.**
03	Pretty Uncharacteristic	**I hardly ever do this.**
02	Quite Uncharacteristic	**I almost never do this.**
01	Extremely Uncharacteristic	**I never do this**

Feedback: Q. No. 2, 3, 6, 9, 10, 12, 14, 16, 18, 20

Exposure: Q. No. 1, 4, 5, 7, 8, 11, 13, 15, 17, 19.

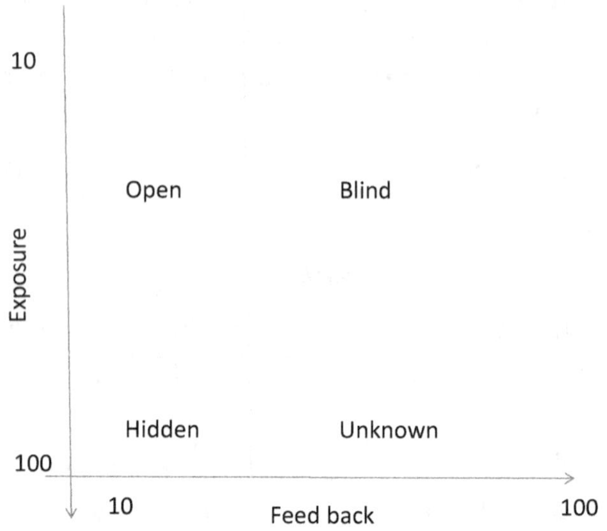

GRAPH

If the : Feed Back total is = 70

Exposure Total is = 80

Conclusion from the graph can be : The Best team building organization

Maslow's hierarchy of needs

Abraham Maslow developed the Hierarchy of Needs model in 1940–50s USA, and the Hierarchy of Needs theory remains valid today for understanding human motivation, management training, and personal development. Indeed, Maslow's ideas surrounding the Hierarchy of Needs concerning the responsibility of employers to provide a workplace environment that encourages and enables employees to fulfill their own unique potential (self-actualization) are today more relevant than ever. Abraham

Maslow's book Motivation and Personality, published in 1954 (second edition 1970) introduced the Hierarchy of Needs, and Maslow extended his ideas in other work, notably his later book "Toward A Psychology Of Being," a significant and relevant commentary, which has been revised in recent times by Richard Lowry, who is in his own right a leading academic in the field of motivational psychology.

Abraham Maslow was born in New York in 1908 and died in 1970, although various publications appear in Maslow's name in later years. Maslow's Ph.D. in psychology in 1934 at the University of Wisconsin formed the basis of his motivational research, initially studying rhesus monkeys. Maslow later moved to New York's Brooklyn College.

The Maslow's Hierarchy of Needs five-stage model below is clearly and directly attributable to Maslow; later versions of the theory with added motivational stages are not so clearly attributable to Maslow. These extended models have instead been inferred by others from Maslow's work. Specifically Maslow refers to the needs Cognitive, Aesthetic and Transcendence as additional aspects of motivation, but not as distinct levels in the Hierarchy of Needs.

Where Maslow's Hierarchy of Needs is shown with more than five levels these models have been extended through interpretation of Maslow's work by other people. These augmented models and diagrams are shown as the adapted seven and eight-stage Hierarchy of Needs pyramid diagrams and models below.

seen.

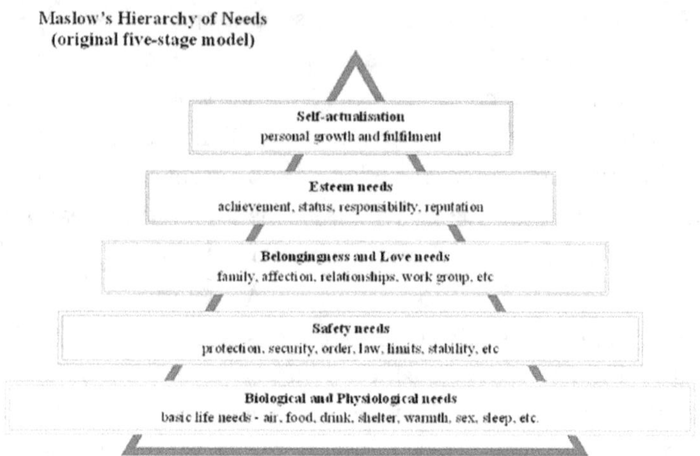

Maslow's hierarchy of needs

Each of us is motivated by needs. Our most basic needs are inborn, having evolved over tens of thousands of years. Abraham Maslow's Hierarchy of Needs helps to explain how these needs motivate us all.

Maslow's Hierarchy of Needs states that we must satisfy each need in turn, starting with the first, which deals with the most obvious needs for survival itself.

Only when the lower order needs of physical and emotional well-being are satisfied are we concerned with the higher order needs of influence and personal development.

Conversely, if the things that satisfy our lower order needs are swept away, we are no longer concerned about the maintenance of our higher order needs.

Maslow's original Hierarchy of Needs model was developed between 1943–1954, and first widely published in Motivation and Personality in 1954. At this time the Hierarchy of Needs model comprised five needs. This original version remains for most people the definitive Hierarchy of Needs.

1. **Biological and Physiological needs** – air, food, drink, shelter, warmth, sex, sleep, etc.

2. **Safety needs** – protection from elements, security, order, law, limits, stability, etc.

3. **Belongingness and Love needs** – work group, family, affection, relationships, etc.

4. **Esteem needs** – self-esteem, achievement, mastery, independence, status, dominance, prestige, managerial responsibility, etc.

5. **Self-Actualization needs** – realizing personal potential, self-fulfillment, seeking personal growth and peak experiences.

This is the definitive and original Maslow's Hierarchy of Needs.

While Maslow referred to various additional aspects of motivation, he expressed the Hierarchy of Needs in these five clear stages.

15. We transact, the way we communicate!

Transactional Analysisis an integrative approach to the theory of psychology and psychotherapy. It is described as integrative because it has elements of psychoanalytic, humanist and cognitive approaches. TA was first developed by Canadian-born US psychiatrist Eric Berne, starting in the late 1950s. According to the International Transactional Analysis Association, TA 'is a theory of personality and a systematic psychotherapy for personal growth and personal change'.

Introduction

All of us are social beings and interact with others in the process of satisfying our human needs and achieving our goals. In management, irrespective of your level, you have to interact with others – peers, superiors and subordinates. And most importantly, in some organizations, with general public. You may have to communicate with people of different sexes, ages, education, skills, personalities and temperaments. Ability to understand the nature and dynamics of interactions with others will help an individual to become more effective communicator – which means more positive respect for self-better performance and achievement of organizational goals, more satisfied and committed employees, effective relationships with superiors and peers, more satisfied consumers or clients.

What is Transactional Analysis? What does T/A do? What does T/A not do? What are the dynamics of T/A? How can I become more effective with the use of T/A?

What is Transactional Analysis?

"Transactional Analysis (T/A) is one of the tools developed by behavioral scientists which is used for analysis of transactions" or understanding of communications that occur between people. It is a rational approach to understanding behavior and is based on the assumption that any person can learn to trust himself or herself, think rationally, make independent decisions, and express feelings. "Transactional Analysis" is a tool but also a complete theory of personality, containing techniques of psychotherapy for personal and social growth. A "transaction" means any exchange or interaction that occurs between two or more persons. Transactional analysis concerns itself with the kinds of communication – both verbal and non-verbal – that occur between people. The emphasis of Transactional Analysis is upon positive communication. Transactional Analysis is widely utilized as a consultation method in educational programmes, social institutions, business, hospitals, churches, government organizations, and other organizations. The late Eric Berne, M.D., the principal innovator and developer of Transactional Analysis, began experimenting with his ideas by applying them to group psychotherapy, but more recently it is widely used in family, couples and individuals work.

What does Transactional Analysis do or not do?

Transactional Analysis increases understanding of self and others. It decreases tendency to be critical of self and others.

Transactional Analysis helps reduces stress, frustration and anxiety levels! A few hours exposure to Transactional Analysis is not necessarily going to result in any person being transformed in to a happy and an effective person. Transactional Analysis does not erase all human relations difficulties. All emotional problems won't be solved with a brief training period and traditional way of doing things that may be non-productive. Lot will depend upon the trainer. There are several who present themselves as experts. These people do more harm than good. Many companies have successfully incorporated Transactional Analysis training in to their overall personnel development programmes. These organizations represent private and public sector industries. State Governments, police systems, educational institutions, municipalities, and professional associations. The benefit which an organization derives from Transactional Analysis are better process diagnosis; clearer problem analysis; reduced non-communication: new tools for selecting people for entry and promotion; and less psychological pollution.

Structural Analysis

According to Transactional Analysis theory, everyone's personality has three parts, called *ego states*. These *ego* states are named *Parent*, *Adult*, and *Child*. When we capitalize these words, we are talking about *ego states* rather than real parents, adults or children. Structural analysis involves analyzing the personality to discover the nature of our ego states. You can use structural analysis to better understand who you are and how you got that way. It will help you learn about the various sources of thoughts, feelings and opinions in your personality. Knowing your personality better can add to your effectiveness on the job.

i) The Parent Ego State

Every one develops a Parent ego state when as children they absorb certain attitudes and ways of behaving from parental figures. When you feel, think, or act as you saw your parents (or other authority figures) act when you were little, you are in your Parent ego state. While in your Parent, you may act in either a controlling, sometimes critical way or in a nurturing, sometimes loving way. Here are some examples of statements you are likely to make while in your Parent.

- **Controlling Parent: "Nobody can leave until this report is finished"**
- **Nurturing Parent: "I'm sorry you're not feeling well today. Would you like to go over to the nurse's office and get some help? I'll take care of your station."**

While in our Parent we respond automatically almost as if a tape recording were playing in our heads and directing our words and actions. For this reason, we often use the phrase "Parent tapes" to refer to:

- Dialogue from Parent figures stored in our heads, and
- Automatic responses we make while in our Parent ego state.

ii) The Adult Ego State

Although we respond automatically when in our Parent, we respond analytically when in our Adult. Whenever you are gathering information, reasoning things out, estimating probabilities, and so on, you are in your Adult ego state. While in this ego state you are cool and collected: you make decisions unemotionally. You just want the facts. The Adult ego state has nothing to do with age. Little children have Adult ego states too! For example, when four-year-old

Vaishali says, "I bet Nikhil is at home – I see his car," she is using her budding Adult, since she is calmly estimating probabilities on the basis of facts.

iii) The Child Ego State

Yes, even though you're an adult, you have a Child inside you. While in your Child ego state, you feel and act like the little person you once were. Your Child has all of the feelings and impulses of a newborn. It also includes your mental recordings of your:

- Early experiences – reactions to these experiences, and – learned view of yourself and other people.

Free or Natural Child (FC or NC)

This is the source of our spontaneity, energy and curiosity, with all our potential for life. It represents the way we are when we are born – natural, loving, carefree, adventurous and trusting – with all our capacities for leading a joyful and meaningful existence. This part of us knows no rules and consequently operates without regard for others and is unconcerned about their reactions. Witness the behavior of the twelve month- old exploring its environment! Of course, it would be impossible to maintain the structure of a society on such a basis, and without some adaptations. In fact, in many grown-ups the adaptations are so extensive that they rarely use their Free Child. Some examples of the expression of the Free Child in an organization are: the joy of a major breakthrough in research and the fun at an office party (alcohol first 'strips away' the Parent, then the Adult!).

Adapted Child

As suggested, it does not seem possible to live in a continuous Free Child state and live with other people at the same time.

From an early age, we make adaptations to help us get along with and get attention from authority figures, most notably our own parents. Some of these may develop in line with general practice in our society, e.g., specific modes of eye and body contact; saying 'please', 'thank you' and 'sorry' at the appropriate times; not making personal comments about others in public. Note how uncomfortable we often feel with those who have not adapted to these culturally agreed ways of behaving. Many more adaptations are unique to the particular family and its situation, and are important in marking us out as individuals. Some examples that create problems in adulthood and are relevant to organizations are compliance, procrastination and rebellion.

Compliance

Some individuals learn when they are young that the way to get along is always to say 'yes'. Their problem in adulthood is saying 'yes' when their better judgment, experience and knowledge suggests that arguing the point and asserting themselves would be more appropriate. Some personal and organizational disasters might have been avoided if some people had not been so compliant in the past. (Of course, some people in power want nothing better than for others to do exactly what they are told!)

Procrastination

Some people learn when they are young that a good way to get attention is to procrastinate. Consider these examples from family life:

Get a move on, or we'll miss the shops!'

'Look, put that doll down, tie your shoe laces up and let's get going.

You're making us late again!'

If a child decides on this basis that delaying gets attention, in adulthood the individual may still be indulging in this behavior. Certainly, being late is a good way to get attention in organizations and it may use up more energy, money and time than it is worth Flextime is no guarantee of cure.

Rebellion

Many children only get attention when they are 'naughty'. Such individuals in adulthood may continue this behavior by seeking bosses and/or institutions (e.g., banks, local government, the police) to constantly fight and rebel against.

Little Professor

Another functional aspect of the Child ego state is frequently introduced and used, although its relationship to the other two is unclear. This is the Little Professor, the intuitive part of us that senses things about other people in a flash. This part of us has those brilliant, non-logical insights giving us solutions to problems that typify some of the major break through in the growth of scientific knowledge.

Transactions and its Analysis

Transactional analysis is related with the way in which individuals interact with each other. It explains the mechanism that takes place when people are having conversation or are trying to exchange their thoughts, feelings and ideas with each other. Thus, Transactional Analysis essentially refers to the analysis of interactions between people. According to Transactional Analysis, transactionsis stimulus plus response (S+R). If two or more people encounter each other, sooner or later one of them will speak, or give some other indication of acknowledging the presence of the others. This is called the "transactional stimulus." Another person will then say or do something which is in some way related to the stimulus, and that is called transaction response. Transactional Analysis involves the study of the social transactions between people and it deals with determining which part of the multiple-natured individual is being activated Parent, Adult or Child.

Transactions and its Types

Normally there are three types of transactions:

    (1) Complementary Transactions;

    (2) Crossed Transactions;

    (3) Ulterior Transactions:

        (a) Duplex;

        (b) Angular

(i) Complementary Transactions

A transaction is complementary when communication continues on parallel lines between individuals and the lines of stimulus and response are parallel. Thus, the message transmitted from one ego-state elicits an expected and appropriate response from the proper ego-state of the other individual. The transactions are complementary because both are acting in the perceived and expected ego-states. Usually, in such a case, both individuals are satisfied, everyone feels OK and the communication is complete. Complementary transactions can take place between

A-A, P-C, P-P and so on.

(ii) Crossed Transactions

The lines of stimulus and Response cross each other in case of crossed transactions. Whenever the stimulus and response cross on the P-A-C transactional diagram, communication stops. Transactions become uncomplimentary. The message sent by one ego-state is responded to from an incompatible, unexpected egostate of another person. The inappropriate response generates feelings of hurt and anger and the individuals, Instead of coming closer, divert from each other. Crossed transactions are the source of much interpersonal conflict in an organization. They inhibit free flow of ideas, free thinking, creativity and social interactions. Crossed transactions have many possible dysfunctional consequences for the organization.

(iii) *Ulterior Transactions*

The ulterior type of transactions are most complex because the communication has double meaning as more than ego-states are involved in them. When ulterior message is sent, the literal and intent meanings are not one and the same. Ulterior message is often disguised in a socially acceptable way. On the surface level, the communication has a clear Adult message, whereas it carries a hidden message on the psychological level. Ulterior transactions like crossed transactions are undesirable as they damage interpersonal relationships.

Strokes

You've seen that transactions can be open, blocked, or ulterior. It's also important to recognize that whenever two people are transacting, they are exchanging "strokes." What are strokes? To help you understand that term, let's look at an important discovery made by Rene Spitz. Spitz found that keeping infants fed and in a clean environment was not enough. Such infants became weak and almost seemed to shrivel up if they were not cuddled and stroked. Infants who are touched very little may become physically and mentally retarded; those not touched at all seem to "give up" and die. Before Spitz discovered this, doctors often puzzled at the high death rate in orphanage nurseries. Today in such nurseries "grandmothers"and "grandfathers" volunteer to come in and just cuddle infants.

In Transactional Analysis language, the term "stroke" refers to the giving of some kind of recognition to a person. This may or may not involve physical touching. As we grow from infancy into childhood and then adulthood, we do not entirely lose our need for stroking. Part of our original need for physical stroking seems to be satisfied with symbolic stroking. We no longer need constant cuddling, but we still need attention. When we receive a stroke, we may choose to feel either good or bad. If we choose to feel good, we might think of the stroke as a "warm fuzzy" (or positive stroke). On the flip side, if we choose to feel bad, we can think of it as a "cold prickly" (or negative stroke).Since we have a basic need for strokes, we will work hard to get them. For example, ignored children will engage in all sorts of creative acts to get stroked. Often such children quickly learn that they can get strokes by:

- Talking in a loud, whiny, high-pitched voice,

- Spilling milk on a clean table cloth, and

- Injuring themselves

A child who carries out one of these actions is likely to get a cold prickly (negative stroke). But it seems to make no difference to a stroke-deprived child. To such a child, any kind of stroke is better than none at all: a cold prickly is better than nothing! The same is true for adults who work in a stroke-deprived environment.

Example

Radhika, a shipping clerk in a small mail-order firm, worked alone. Yet she got a lot of strokes from Sushil, her supervisor. Sushil often stopped by Radhika's work station just to chat. These strokes were not usually given for any particular job performance since Radhika's job was rather routine and didn't require any special skills. However, Sushil did compliment Radhika for his consistent performance. Then one day Sushil was promoted. Radhika's new supervisor, Manali, had a different approach. Shedidn't stop to chat with her subordinates and spoke to them only when she was dissatisfied with their work.

Life positions

Another way of looking at relationships between people is through the concept of 'life position', sometimes referred to as the basic position or existential position. A person's life position at any given time expresses in some way just how that individual is relating to others in terms of thinking, feeling and behaving.

There are four basic life positions, shown below referred to as the OK corral.

Examples of Life Positions

The idea of life positions can be demonstrating the following examples.

1. 'Hey, we did a good job there', says the boss.

'Yes, things are really going well for us now', says the subordinate.

(I'm OK, you're OK)

2. 'Your work is not up to the standard I need in this department!' says the boss.

(I'm OK, you're not OK)

3. 'I wish I could keep on top of things the way you can', says the subordinate.

(I'm not OK, you're OK)

4. 'Well, I don't know what to do and you don't know what to do. What a mess!' says the boss.

(I'm not OK, you're not OK)

Characteristics of the Life Positions:

I'M OK, YOU'RE OK (I + U+)

This is sometimes referred to as the **get on** *with* position. People occupying this position are optimistic, confident and happy about work and life. They use time constructively, doing the things they most want to. They exchange strokes freely with those they meet, accepting the significance of other people, and decline to put themselves or others down. They are assertive in reaching their aims, i.e., they state and elaborate their own views and needs rather than attack other people's views and needs. Their dominant working style with others is collaboration and mutual respect, sharing authority and responsibility and listening constructively, even if they disagree. The problems they encounter in work and life are faced and dealt with as constructively as possible. They are likely to 'succeed' in life within the limits they've set themselves, finding satisfaction with work and relationships, and tend to live long, healthy lives.

I'M OK, YOU'RE NOT OK (I+ U-)

This is sometimes referred to as the **get rid** *of* position. It is characterized by feelings of anger, fury and hostility. Others are seen as inferior, unworthy, incompetent, wrong and not to be trusted. Behavior too thers is characterized by such things as spite, victimization, trapping, condescension, abuse and disregard. They may devote much time to the destruction of the sense of self-worth of others. As well as putting others down, they over-inflate their own self-worth, deny personal problems and find it difficult to give positive strokes. At work they are highly competitive and climb over others at whatever cost to achieve power and status. In wider social terms this is the life position of those who exploit their fellow man, or of those who take dogmatic views, believing theirs to be the only right course. In extreme cases they are homicidal (You are so "not OK," there's no point to your living')

I'M NOT OK, YOU'RE OK (I- U+)

This is referred to as the **get away from** position and is typified by feelings such as sadness, inadequacy, stupidity or a sense of being ugly. In this position, people experience themselves as inferior or powerless in relation to others. They put themselves down and find it difficult to accept positive strokes, even being suspicious of them. In relation to work, they undervalue their potential and skills and they avoid or with draw from difficult situations and problems. In life generally, they don't succeed, are unhappy, often ill and/or depressed and in extreme cases commit suicide (I'm so useless I may as well not live')

I'M NOT OK, YOU'RE NOT OK (I- U-)

This is also referred to as the **get nowhere position** and is accompanied by feelings of confusion or aimlessness and pointlessness. Their attitude is 'Why bother, what's the point?' and they frequently waste time. They do nothing very much in life, and in extreme cases become alcoholics or drug addicts, or go crazy, possibly committing murder or suicide.

Summary:
Why do we transact?

1. Better process diagnosis of the problem.
2. Clearer problem analysis.
3. Reduce Non Communication.
4. New tool for selecting people for entry.
5. Less psychological pollution.

Because we are social beings!

1. Social beings interact with others in the process of satisfying Our human needs and achieving goals.
2. Irrespective of your level, you have to interact with others – peers,Superiors and subordinates and general public.
3. You communicate with different sexes, ages, education, skills, personalities and temperaments.

Transactional analysis helps:

1. Ability to understand the nature and dynamics of interaction With others will help an individual to become more effective communicator.
2. Positive approach.
3. Better performance.
4. More satisfied employees, consumers or clients.
5. Effective relationship with all stake holders.
6. Increases understanding of self and others.

7. Decreases tendency to be critical of self and others.

8. Helps reduce stress, frustration and anxiety levels.

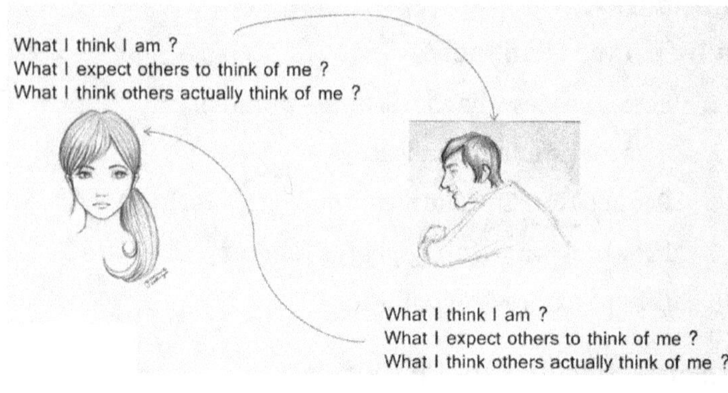

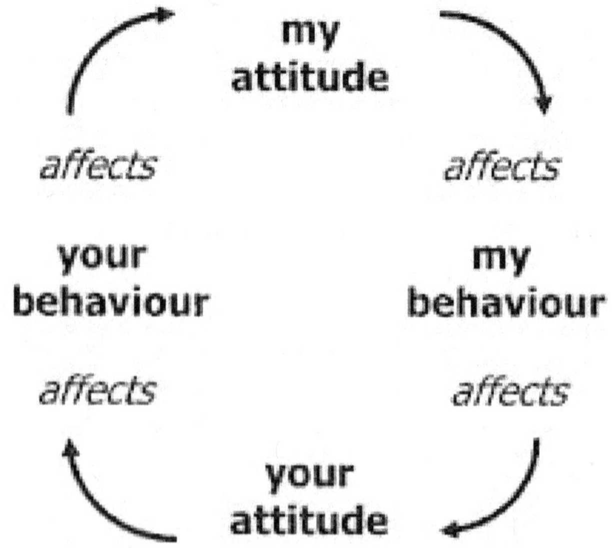

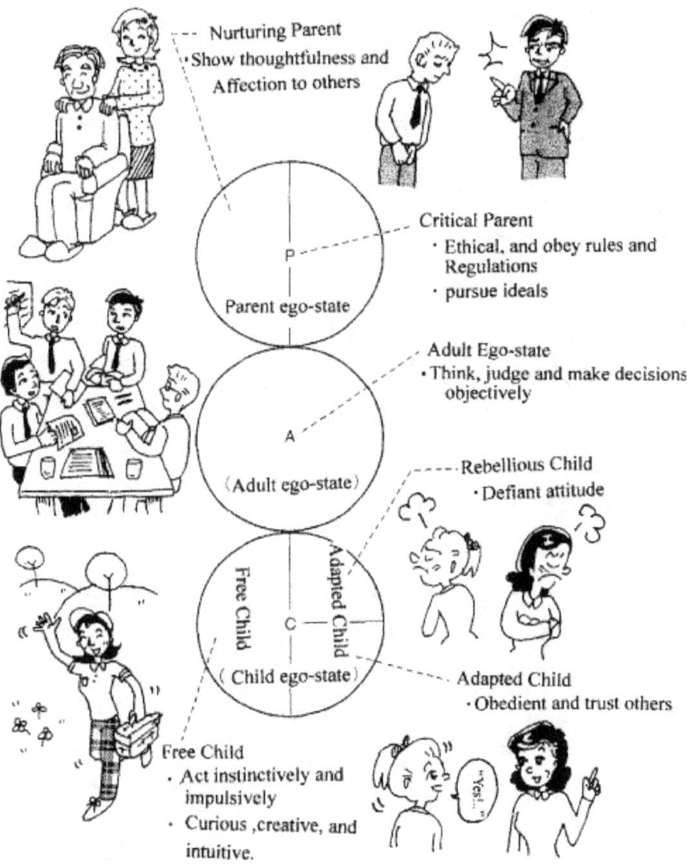
Nurturing Parent
Show thoughtfulness and
Affection to others
Critical Parent
Ethical, and obey rules and
Regulations
pursue ideals
P
Parent ego-state
Adult Ego-state
Think, judge and make decisions
objectively
A
(Adult ego-state)
Rebellious Child
Defiant attitude
Free Child
Adapted Child
C
(Child ego-state)
Adapted Child
Obedient and trust others
Free Child
Act instinctively and
impulsively
Curious, creative, and
intuitive.
"Yes!"

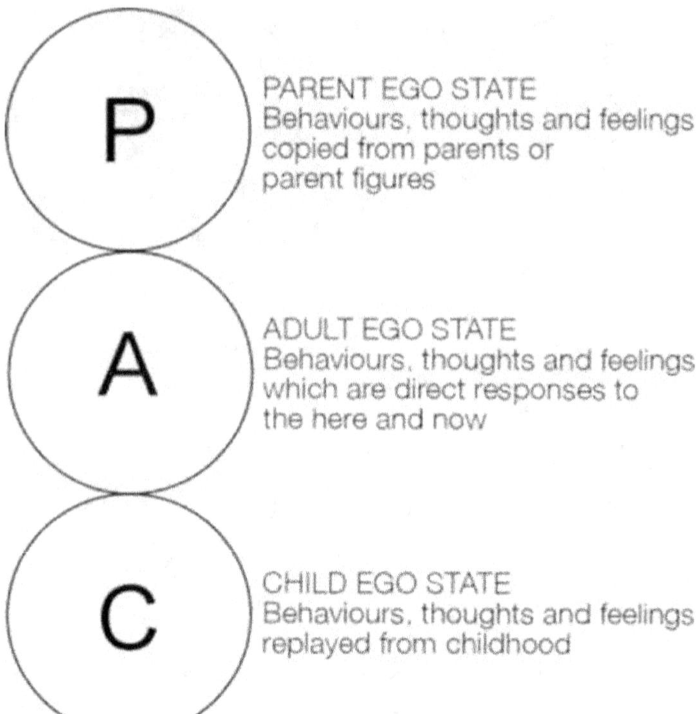

P
PARENT EGO STATE
Behaviours, thoughts and feelings
copied from parents or
parent figures
A
ADULT EGO STATE
Behaviours, thoughts and feelings
which are direct responses to
the here and now
C
CHILD EGO STATE
Behaviours, thoughts and feelings
replayed from childhood

16. Are you ready for the change?

Outdoor Based Experiential Training involves the presentation of meaningful change in to the people within the framework of safety, in order to give them a deep personal and social awareness. Here situations being Unknown, Real, Unforeseen and Novel, they promote an individual to change and think differently. This will bring desired change happen effectively.

You must be the change you wish to see in the world. Everybody wants to change, but when it comes to reality, nobody wants to change. Why? You want others to change first. Even the people who say that they need and love change, can be stressed by it after a certain point. Most of us spend much of our lives waiting for someone else to change so we will be happier, free and more successful.

Do you know friends! "Change Management" – this word has four **grammatical** facets as follows.

It's a noun: "***Change management*** is key to the project."

It's a verb: "We really need to ***change manage*** that process."

It's an adjective: "My ***change management*** skills are improving."

It's an expletive: "***Change management!***"

But what exactly is it?

Change management is a structured approach for ensuring that changes are thoroughly and smoothly implemented, and that the lasting benefits of change are achieved. It is making organization change effectively.

The change management process is the sequence of steps or activities that a change management team or project leader would follow to apply change management to a project or change. Based on Prosci's research of the most effective and commonly applied change, they have created a change management process that contains the following three phases:

Phase 1 – Preparing for change (Preparation, assessment and strategy development)

Phase 2 – Managing change (Detailed planning and change management implementation)

Phase 3 – Reinforcing change™ (Data gathering, corrective action and recognition)

Defining change management

It is important to note what change management is and what change management is not, as defined by the majority of research participants.

- Change management *is not* a stand-alone process for designing a business solution.
- Change management *is* the processes, tools and techniques for managing the people-side of change.
- Change management *is not* a process improvement method.
- Change management *is* a method for reducing and managing resistance to change when implementing process, technology or organizational change.
- Change management *is not* a stand-lone technique for improving organizational performance.

- Change management *is* a necessary component for any organizational performance improvement process to succeed, including programs like: Six Sigma, Business Process Reengineering, Total Quality Management, Organizational Development, Restructuring an continuous process improvement.

- Change management *is* how we drive the adoption and usage we need to realize business results.

Prosci's definition of change management: Change management is the application of a structured process and set of tools for leading the people – side of change to achieve a desired outcome. Prosci surveyed more than 3400 organizations over the last 15 years. According to him there are eight elements comprise the areas or components of a change management program.

Components of Change Management:

1. Readiness Assessments:

Assessments are tools used by a change management team or project leader to assess the organization's readiness to change. Readiness assessments can include, organizational assessments, culture and history assessments, employee assessments, sponsor assessments and change assessments. Each tool provides the project team with insights into the challenges and opportunities they may face during the change process.

- Assess the scope of the change, including: How big is this change? How many people are affected? Is it a gradual or radical change?

- Assess the readiness of the organization impacted by the change, including: What is the value- system and background of the impacted groups? How much change is already going on? What type of resistance can be expected?

- Assess the strengths of your change management team.

- Assess the change sponsors and take the first steps to enable them to effectively lead the change process.

2. Communication and communication planning

Many managers assume that if they communicate clearly with their employees, their job is done. However, there are many reasons why employees may not hear or understand what their managers are saying the first time around. In fact, you may have heard that messages need to be repeated 6 to 7 times before they are cemented into the minds of employees. That is because each employee's readiness to hear depends on many factors. Effective communicators carefully consider three components: the audience, what is said and when it is said. For example, the first step in managing change is building awareness around the need for change and creating a desire among employees. Therefore, initial communications are typically designed to create awareness around the business reasons for change and the risk of not changing. Likewise, at each step in the process, communications should be designed to share the right messages at the right time.

Communication planning, therefore, begins with a careful analysis of the audiences, key messages and the timing for those messages. The change management team or project leaders must design a communication plan that addresses the needs of front-line employees, supervisors and executives.

Each audience has particular needs for information based on their role in the implementation of the change.

3. Sponsor activities and sponsor road maps:

Business leaders and executives play a critical sponsor role in change management. The change management team must develop a plan for sponsor activities and help key business leaders carry out these plans. Sponsorship should be viewed as the most important success factor. Avoid confusing the notion of sponsorship with support. The CEO of the company may support your project, but that is not the same as sponsoring your initiative.

Sponsorship involves active and visible participation by senior business leaders throughout the process which can be effectively implemented through OBET. Unfortunately many executives do not know what this sponsorship looks like. A change agent's or project leader's role includes helping senior executives do the right things to sponsor the project.

4. Coaching and manager training for change management

Supervisors will play a key role in managing change. Ultimately, the direct supervisor has more influence over an employee's motivation to change than any other person at work. Unfortunately, supervisors as a group can be the most difficult to convince of the need for change and can be a source of resistance. It is vital for the change management team and executive sponsors to gain the support of supervisors and to build change leadership. Individual change management activities should be used to help these supervisors through the change process.

Once managers and supervisors are on board, the change management team must prepare a coaching strategy. They will need to provide training for supervisors including how to use individual change management tools with their employees.

5. Training and training development

Training is the cornerstone for building knowledge about the change and the required skills. Project team members will develop training requirements based on the skills, knowledge and behaviors necessary to implement the change. These training requirements will be the starting point for the training group or the project team to develop training programs. Identifying a proper service provider or a trainer based on your requirements play a key role in ultimate success.

6. Resistance management

Resistance from employees and managers is normal. Persistent resistance, however, can threaten a project. The change management team needs to identify, understand and manage resistance throughout the organization. Resistance management is the processes and tools used by managers and executives with the support of the project team to manage employee resistance.

7. Data collection, feedback analysis and corrective action

Employee involvement is a necessary and integral part of managing change. Managing change is not a one way street. Feedback from employees is a key element of the change management process. Analysis and corrective action based on this feedback provides a robust cycle for implementing change.

8. Celebrating and recognizing success

Early successes and long-term wins must be recognized and celebrated. Individual and group recognition is also a necessary component of change management in order to cement and reinforce the change in the organization. The final step in the change management process is the after-action review. It is also known as Evaluation. It is at this point that you can stand back from the entire program, evaluate successes and failures, and identify process changes for the next project. This is part of the ongoing, continuous improvement of change management for your organization and ultimately leads to change competency.

These eight elements comprise the areas or components of a change management program. You need to look beyond, you need to look in to the future to crystallize the vision. [**Model 1.**] Along with the change management process, they create a system for managing change. Good project managers apply these components effectively to ensure project success, avoid the loss of valued employees, and minimize the negative impact of the change on productivity and a company's customers

Most of the people go through Four natural stages when change comes to reality.

Example: When the computers were introduced in India by Late Priminister Rajeev Gandhi.

1. **Denial:** I do not believe that this change is necessary or that will work.

2. **Resistance**: I absolutely refuse to do as I have been instructed in light of the change.

3. **Exploration:** I want to learn more about the change, review the pros and cons and determine the implications of the change.

4. **Acceptance**: I think this change is working, as I think about it, I even think it makes a lot of sense.

How to increase your ability to change?

1. Choose Differently:

This begins with knowing that you choose to be where you are right now professionally and personally, and you choose your current work attitudes and life style. So you always choose more positive attitudes towards the necessary transitions in your life.

2. Ask for Help:

Have a humility and willingness to ask for the help you need. You are not expected to know everything. So read a book, Hire a consultant, take a course. Then take daily responsibilities for current choices and new results.

3. Hurt enough or Change:

"Invite pains and postpone pleasures." Former addicts call this "HITTING BOTTOM".

If the life you are now leading has any pain in it, that pain is usually a good motivator to cause you to look at thinking, being and doing differently. When you are sufficiently uncomfortable, you might be ready to use next key.

4. Never Quit:

Negative thoughts and beliefs are often part of mindset. So you must keep on *One day, One idea, One change* at a time.

5. **Grab on to the New, Let go off the old:**

Letting go is harder than hanging on. For change to be real and lasting, you must make a decision, a commitment, to let go of your old ways of thinking, doing and being and relating.

6. **Embrace a New way:**

Find some joy in it to persist. It is just like starting an aerobic or an exercise programme. Find actions and attitudes you truly enjoy, so you will be able to continue enthusiastically for more than three weeks...21 days is a time it takes to install a new habit. It is your responsibility to make the new way as positive as possible for yourself and your dependants.

7. **Stop playing Victims:**

Do not blame the past, present and future or whomsoever else you want to blame. Do not blame the environment around. No one did this for you. Serve others, surround yourself with positive supportive people and be a creator.

So learn to Choose more positive attitude towards life, Take daily responsibilities, When you are uncomfortable, be ready to use next key., Keep one day, one idea, one change at a time and Do not blame the past, look at the future.

Hence Change is the only constant: Bring the change in to your

1. Policy [Autonomy, ISO]

2. Culture [Liberalization, Privatization, Globalizationin business]

3. Arrangements [Unforeseen situation]

4. Beliefs [Do not brand the people, Institutions and events etc.]

5. Methodology [Inductive]

6. Mindset [Ego]

7. Life style [Healthy life style like Morning walk etc.]

8. Attitude [Social]

9. Situation [Things happen differently in similar situation]

10. Working style [Multimedia, I T, Eco-friendly]

Every organization is in need of flexible people who can accept and adopt changes swiftly, because changes are inevitable. Changes make life more interesting and challenging. Without understanding this, we suffer, complain, get frustrated and try to shift the responsibility of our ignorance on somebody else when changes transpire. Change may be accelerating a hidden blessing. The best principle when circumstances change is "You Change." Handling change and successfully managing it is an art, a tactful skill, quite interestingly it can be learnt. We have to change our thinking habits. New thoughts will lead a person to be filled with great amount of positive attitude, energy and enthusiasm that is essential to manage the change.

A crucial factor of the universe is that it changes continuously. Therefore change is always there, whether you accept it or not, whether you stay happy in a changed circumstance or not. Some people fail to sustain and manage the change because they lack desire, determination and confidence to revert the changed environment to their favor.

According to Huge Downs "A happy person is not a person in a certain set of circumstances, but rather a person with a certain set of attitudes." That attitude is to change when circumstances change. It is said life is collection of changes; every change is a challenge and challenge when faced may bring success Or else they may act as stepping –stone to success.

Art of managing the change:

The process of change starts from "Thinking" [**Refer Model 2.**] When you change your **Thinking,** you change your **Belief** ; When you change your **Belief,** you change your **Behavior** ; When you change your **Behavio**r, you change your **Attitude**; When you change your **Attitude,** you change your **Performance** ; When you change your **Performance,** you change your **Life.** So if you really want to change your life, Always know and be prepared that change is inevitable, Expect and accept the change, Handle the change without burdening your mind and anxiety, enjoy the change, Take a responsibility to be happy, grow from the change and Be ready and expect a new change.

Rational thinking tells you the way to Change:

Example: My daily local trains travel in Mumbai.

1. **Events are impersonal and indifferent:** People travel in Local Trainwith different moods. But the travel is impersonal and Indifferent.

2. **Men are disturbed not by the Things but by the views they take of them:** I am disturbed because in my view, I wanted No rains, no crowd, no waste of time etc. during my Local travel.

3. **Understand what you can control And what you cannot:**I was exaggerating the overcrowding Local

Train situation. In fact I must learn to pass my time effectively because Local Travel is like that only.

4. **After all, freedom is something Chosen, not given:** I do not have any alternative to Travel by Local train. I have chosen this mode of travel, So I must Change my attitude and think rational.

5. **Is it an emotional death where I cease to be a human?** I have become used to this travel. Having known that any fetal accident can happen during this travel, I am travelling in Local train. I have Lost the emotions. I have just become a machine this is my emotional death.

6. **Reason is supreme:** Stop playing victims. Do not blame the past. Convert the calamity into Opportunity. Accept the fact.

Remember! Never change the value system!

We do not have control over the events happening, but certainly we can choose how to deal with them. It is always better and smarter to manage change with a positive mindset. Rather than being reactive. we can be proactive and develop authentic thinking, wherein we can judge, analyze and decide. We should change as per changes in life, but there are few things which should not change – that is our value system- values like integrity, commitment, honesty and loyalty. If values are dead in a man then nothing in the world can revive and reinstate his existence.Changes are nothing beyond human endurance. We should learn to treat changes occurring in our lives with equanimity. Welcome change with enthusiasm. It keeps us alive.

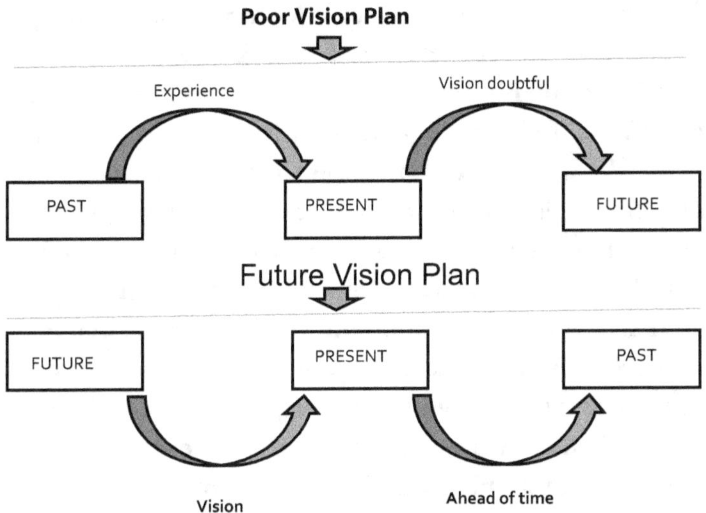

Model 1:Future Vision Plan for Effective Change Management

This model gives you two plans. The upper is the Poor vision plan. It starts from the past experiences. Management gurus say that man hardly learns from the past experience. Therefore we never should decide the Present based on the past experience. Things shall never happen the same way in the similar situations in future. We assume many wrong things based on the past experience. So we wrongly decide our present and of course based on the wrong assumptions we try to plan our future strategies. It gives poor vision. It can at the most decide the short time strategy only.

Examples: No need to go for multiple marriages, to learn how to be a good spouse or No need to wait until your last child has grown, to master parenthood.

The lower part of the model is future vision plan which starts from the Future itself and ends in to the past...

Look beyond yourself. Learn from the experience you get out of an event. Try to visualize the future of that event. Think thoroughly, apply your creative mind and decide what kindof changes in the existing plan are necessary to decide the present short term strategy. Appoint a team of futurologists to decide the Long term strategy to be adopted in the coming future. So Future vision plan takes you ahead of time through Long term strategy. In this plan your strategies are so pinpointed that as per the plan you go on completing the tasks well in time and put them in to past. More faster you will be putting the tasks in to the past, more effective will be your Change and Time management. Patience in planning and Impatience in execution can make wonders!

Example: Resistance to our National policy of Computerization! Those who had a future vision, adopted it immediately. Majority of Indian human resource in service sector resisted it for long 15 years.

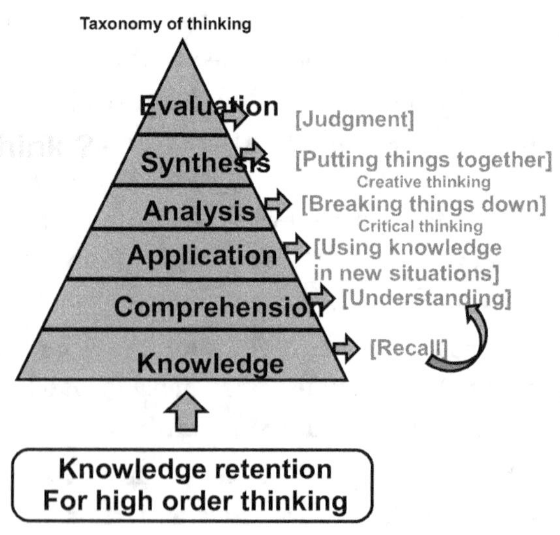

Model 2: How to think? is more important than What to think?

Originality in thinking or indigenous thinking is the outcome of Creativity or innovation. This type of approach to thinking is possible only if we learn How to think? Knowledge is the base of high order thinking. When we filter out the noise [unwanted] from Information, it becomes a knowledge. As a result of learning, have you really understood the core facts? So you must comprehend the knowledge. If you don't, better recall the Knowledge. Once you have understood, then use that knowledge in to new situation. This is where you try to Apply the knowledge. After Application of the knowledge, analyze it Critically. Critical analysis is done by breaking and sequencing the overall application in to smaller applications. This type of thinking is known as Critical thinking. Once you have critically analyzed it, try to put the things together again. You can try it out with different permutation combinations. This is known as Synthesis. Synthesis requires Creative thinking. Now the Idea or the Pilot model, or the machine, or the process or the service or the technology whatever you have developed, is put to test through the process of Evaluation. This Evaluation gives you judgment about the product. Now your wisdom of judging the product will ultimately decide the acceptance or rejection of the new product. This is how an effective change is brought about. At any step, if your understanding is not 100%, better recall the previous step and try to understand it thoroughly.

So in the mathematical language of "Thinking" the equation is "100-1 = 0"

References:

Barker, D., TA and Training, *Gower Publishing Company Ltd.*, 1982.

Broderick, R. "Learning the Ropes," *Training,* October 1989.

Cosgrove, D. J., "The outdoor Experience," Midwest Academy of Management meeting, Toledo, Ohio, April 1988.

Chris Bonington, "Everest the hard way," *Vikas Publishing House Pvt. Ltd.*, 23 December 1976.

E. Berne, "Games People Play," *Grove Press Inc.*, 1964; Penguin, 1968.

Ewert, A.W. *"Outdoor Adventure Pursuits: Foundation, Models and Theories,"* Columbus, Ohio: Publishing Horizons.

Falvey, Jack, "Before spending $3 Million on Leadership, Read this "*Wall Street Journal,* October 3, 1988.

Galagan, Patricia, "Between two Trapezes." *Training and Development Journal,* March 1987.

Galagan, Patricia, "Execs Go Global, Literally.," *Training and Development Journal,* June 1990.

Gall, Adrienne, "You can take the Managers out of the woods, but ...," *Training and Development Journal,* March 1987.

Garvey, D. "The corporate connection: From Bowlines to Bowties" *The Journal of Experimental Education,* 1989.

Hundley, W. "Overcoming obstacles to Trust,"*Dayton Obio Daily News,* January 6, 1990.

John Bank, "Outdoor development for Managers.," *Gower Publishing Company Ltd.*, 1982.

Latteier, C. "Learning to Lead." *US Air*, 1989.

Long, J. W., The wilderness Lab Comes of Age *"Training and Development Journal*, March 1987.

MacNeil-Lehrer Productions, "Focus Upword Bound," *MacNeil-Lehrer Newshour television broadcast, New York: WNET Television*, September 4, 1990.

McEvoy, Glenn M, and Paul F. Buller. "Five Uneasy Pieces in the Training Evaluation Puzzle," *Training and Development Journal*, August 1990.

Mumford, A., "What's News in Management Development?" *Personnel Management*, May 1985.

Petrini Catherine, "Over the Rivers and Through the woods,"*Training and Development Journal*, May 1990.

Ranjan Garge, "Mountaineering," *Saket Prakashan*, 1994.

Roland Christopher, "Transfer of Outdoor Managerial Training to the Workplace." Unpublished dissertation, 1981.

Ronald Christopher, S, Summers, M, Friedman, G, Barton and K, McCarthy, "Creation of an Experimental Challenge programme.," *Therapeutic Recreation Journal*," Volume 21, Number 2, 1987.

Schoel, J., and R, Prouty. *Islands of Healing*. Hamilton, Massachusetts: Project Adventure, 1988.

Seligson, T. "To survive We must Trust," *Parade*, October 8, 1989.

"Welcome to Hell Camp." *Time*, March 7, 1989.

Wells K. "The authentic approach from Quarterbacks' Motivational talks to Rock climbing. Programmes Promote Risk taking for Executives," *Wall Street Journal*, September 3, 1988.

Wolman,R. "Training among the Trees" *Northeast Training News*, 1981.

Zemke,Ron. "Personal Growth Training," *Training*, May 1978.

www.ingramcontent.com/pod-product-compliance
Lightning Source LLC
Chambersburg PA
CBHW051736250726
48659CB00001B/99

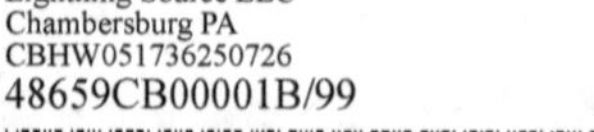